Ceridwen's Handbook of Incense Oils and Candles

Being a guide to the magickal and spiritual uses of oils, incense, candles and the like

by Maya Heath

Cover art by Steve Goins

Typesetting and Illustrations by Wade Berlin

Merlyn Press
630 South Huttig
Independence, MO 64053

Ceridwen's Handbook of Incense Oils and Candles

Copyright © 1996 Robert B. Isaac

All rights reserved. No part of the contents of this book may be reproduced in any form or by any means without the written permission of the publisher.

Published in the United States by Merlyn Press

Manufactured in the United States of America

ISBN 0-9651554-0-4

Statement of Copyright

All recipes and formula names appearing in this work are the property of Ceridwen's Magical, Metaphysical & New Age Supplies and may not be copied or used in any way, except by express written permission. Ceridwen's Handbook of Incense Oils and Candles © 1996 Robert B. Isaac. All parts reserved, no part of this publication may be reproduced by any means or in any way whatsoever without written permission from the publisher, except for brief quotations embodied in literary articles or reviews. Some Interior Illustrations Copyright 1996 Wade Berlin, Portions Copyright 1996 Ancient Pathways Corp., used with Permission. Some Interior Illustrations are from "The Complete Encyclopedia of Illustration " by J.G. Heck, copyright © Crown Publishers and are used with permission.

all things exist within divine order

an it harm none, do what thou wilt,
shall be the whole of the law

Acknowledgments

A project of this magnitude cannot be accomplished alone. Although one pen may write the words, many hands are needed to bring those words into a finished work.

I am deeply grateful to my family and friends for their continued love and support through this project, and to Bob Isaac for his support and encouragement. Many thanks and deep appreciation goes to Nick Nuessle for his invaluable technical assistance when all seemed lost. To Sandra Roberson for her patient and careful editing. And especially to Wade Berlin who brought this whole project from potential to reality with both his extraordinary creative talent and technical expertise. I would like to thank Steve Goins for the cover art. My thanks to Timothy Morefield of Wax Dragon Candle Co. in St Louis, Mo for his valuable input in the discussion of sympathetic magic using various candle shapes.

This book is dedicated to Ed Peach and Sybil Leek who laid its foundation for me.

Contents

Acknowledgments 5
The Cottage in the Wood 8
The Power of Fragrance 11
Essential Oils 12
    The Powers of Essential Oils 14
    The Harmonies of Fragrance 22
The Elements of Magick 23
Creating a Universe 25
    The Essence Portrait 25
Air 27
    Incense 27
Fire 29
    Candles 29
    In The Light 30
    The Shape of Your Candles 31
    Preparing Your Candles 33
    A Simple Candle Spell 33
Water 34
    Bath Crystals 34
Earth 36
    The Energies of Stones 37
Spirit 41
Tarot 43
    Major Arcana Symbology 43
Working by the Stars 45
    Planetary Attributes Chart 47
    Astrological Candles & Oils 48
    Timing Your Work by the Planets 50
    Planetary Hour Charts 50
    The Moon's Influence 51
    Your magickal wish spell 52
Magickal Blends 56
Ritual 77
    Ritual Formulas 77
    Celebrations & Sabbats 79

Healing & Transformation 80
   The Magick of Color 80
   Your Inner Rainbow 80
   Chakras 82
   Chakra Healing & Strengthening Process 84
The Universe of Spirit & Archetypes 85
   Spiritual Magick 87
Spiritual Formulas 89
   African Powers 89
   Angels 90
   Enochian 91
   Tree of Life (Kaballah) 92
   Arthurian 93
   Assyro-Babylonian Deities 95
   British and Celtic Deities 96
   Christian 97
   Egyptian Deities And Essences 98
   Hindu Deities and Legendary Persons 102
   Mythical Creatures 106
   Mythical Places 106
   Norse Deities and Legendary Persons 107
   Greco-Roman Deities and Legendary Persons 110
   Oriental Wisdom 113
   Shamanic 114
   Shamanic Essential Fragrances 116
   Welsh Deities and Legendary Persons 117
   Wiccan Archetypes 119
Bibliography 121
About the Author 123
About the Cover Artist 123
About Ceridwen's 124
   Ceridwen's Magickal & New Age Supplies 125
   Copyright Notice 125

The Cottage in the Wood

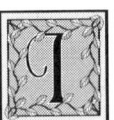

I had walked since first light from the village beyond the wood and it was nearly dark when I came to the old woman's door. They had told me the wise woman lived there, whispering that she was a witch who dealt with forbidden things. But, they had also told in stronger tones how she could cool a fever, or treat a festering wound with a poultice made of herbs, so I knew she was the one I sought. I had come such a long way to get here and I was so tired, but as I knocked on her door my mind was blank. What would I say to her? How could I ask for what I needed? What ailed me was something so much deeper than a poultice could ever draw. My fever was of the heart, not the body.

I heard the bolt draw aside, the hinges protesting as the door was drawn back. Then, she stood there silhouetted by the firelight, a bent shape in a shawl. Without a word she moved aside motioning me to enter. As I stepped across the threshold into the warmth of the fire-lit room, I saw herbs hanging in bundles from hooks set in the heavy wooden rafters, saw jars on ranks of shelves against the wall, saw the small iron cauldron simmering on a hook over the fire, smelled the rich heady aroma of the place. After the cold and dark of the forest it made my head swim a little and I drew a deep breath to savor the countless fragrances. With a gesture she motioned me to a seat by the fire, then drew her own seat and sat confronting me.

"And what brings you so far from home?" She asked. It was not the cracked voice of the crone I had expected, but rich and deep, full of intelligence and power. "To have walked all this way, you cannot be ailing. You are young, perhaps a charm to bring you luck in life? Perhaps to bring you the love of one who does not see you? Perhaps to bring vengeance on a rival?"

There was laughter in her voice, a kind of mockery that told me she knew I came for none of these things - nothing so simple. My voice had left me and I could only shake my head. The time had come to speak, but I had lost the words for what I wanted more than anything in the world. I drew a breath, I raised my head, and then my eyes met hers. And such eyes they were in such a face. A thousand years looked back at me in humor and in strength. Eyes the color of moss, of peat, of night, of morning. She was ageless old, her features shaped by all the years and by knowledge such as I could only imagine, but beautiful as few women dream of. There was such wisdom there, such compassion, such perception. Those eyes looked into my soul and suddenly my tongue was free because I knew she had already discerned the purpose of my quest.

"I want to know." I said. "I want to know about these things here. About the herbs and the healing and the things beyond all that. I want to know what the root does in secret in the earth and what the stars do in fire in the void. I came all this way and I want to know." Those ageless beautiful eyes knew my heart, knew the hunger there. In that moment before she spoke I have never been so afraid. I feared that she would set me out the door, deny my search and close her door. I could not bear that. I had come so far. But she laughed instead, a laugh that held the warmth of a thousand summer suns and the joy of a thousand springtime mornings.

"Yes, you have come a long way indeed." She chuckled "And you have a great hunger there inside you. But like the starving man you cannot have it all at once. You must find out first how to learn these things you want so badly. You must find the first teachers. You must start with simple things - the things closest to you like your body. What does your body tell you? Do you even know? What does your nose tell you about this place? Your nose is the doorway to your inner self. It talks to your instincts and your other senses long before it ever talks to your brain. You remember with your nose. You taste with it. It tells you things that you have no words for. It triggers the impulses sleeping inside you. You see, humans are also animals, child, animals with noses with instincts. One smell can make you happy, another can make you quiet, still another can make you fall in love. Smells can strengthen the heart or make you sleep. Yes, just a smell. Something you can't even see.

"What else does this scent do as it surrounds you? It is there, you know, even though you cannot see it. It is there like the wind, like the morning light. It touches you all over, does it not, like the wind. Invisible, it touches your skin all over your body. And what does it do then? Why, your skin drinks it in. Did you think that all your skin did was keep your bones from falling apart? No child, your skin breathes by itself. With a thousand tiny mouths it drinks the air around you. With your sweat it cleanses the poisons from you. Your skin touches the world in a thousand ways. It is your connection to everything around you. What else does this scent do, besides enter your heart through your nose and your body through your skin? Why, the very energy around you changes because of it. The life currents of your body move with it and change because of it. So powerful is this thing you cannot even see. Now this is what you want to know. How do we harness this powerful and invisible thing? How do we use it to heal, to hearten and to change? Where does its spirit rest that we can find it and waken it to our purpose?"

She reached upward to where a bunch of dried plants hung in the shadows above us. Her ancient hands were graceful as birds. Her practiced and skillful fingers twisted a leaf from the dried and withered branch. She brought it close to my face and crushed it beneath my nose. Instantly my heart lightened. The fatigue of the journey that had dragged so heavily only a moment before lifted and the soreness in my muscles began to release. She chuckled again enjoying the joke and my wonder at it.

"Yes, even when it looks so dead as though there could not be an ounce of life left in it. There it is still - sleeping - waiting for us to call on it when we need. Such a little thing, a leaf and nothing more, or it might have been a flower, or perhaps a root." She gestured again and I saw other bundles, some with withered petals hanging down along with their faded foliage. There on the shelf I saw jars holding bundles of brown gnarled sticks. This is what I had come for. I knew it now. But how did it work? What was this power that hid so skillfully in such unassuming things? She saw the wonder in my eyes. She must have felt my heart longing for it in the stillness between us because she laughed again, her eyes dancing in the firelight winked with green and gold lights.

"You know that the plants move with the seasons. Yes, you know all that. Anyone knows that. But who can know how else they move? They are rooted in the very earth itself. What else do they drink through those roots besides moisture from the rain? They take in the life of the earth, the pulse of it, the power of it. Their very lives are the song of the days, the seasons. Their life and death are all of one piece with the clockwork of the universe. They turn with the sun's light, they grow with the moon's tides. They sing the song of the planets and the elemental currents of the earth. They take these powers, these forces and weave them into their own special song - each kind so different from the rest . They take all these forces and bind them into their innermost natures, distill them into the oils that hold them, some in the leaf, or flower or branch or root. They hide them well, their powers woven from the song of the world and the universe it moves through. You see, child, when you know the plants, you'll know the larger world. They'll tell you; they'll teach you, but, first, you must know how to listen. That's why you've come. And I think you'll stay awhile. There's work here for you."

She took my hand then and opened it. On my open palm she dusted the fragments of the leaf she had crushed. So simple - so infinite.

The Power of Fragrance

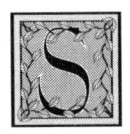

Scents and smells form an invisible molecular cloud that surrounds your whole body. The sensory apparatus of your nose reacts to the scent molecules by triggering thousands of microscopic chemical reactions that carry messages to the brain. Every odor you perceive whether pleasant or noxious, causes minute chemical reactions in your brain causing a reaction whether you are conscious of it or not. You know when food is rotten or a flower is sweet. You breathe in the multitude of forest fragrances or inhale deeply of the sea air. You sniff the kitchen for cookies or pot roast. Each of these smells carries many messages, some conscious and some much deeper. You react to smells on many levels, in many ways. They affect your memory and your subconscious, triggering your instincts rather than your conscious reactions. Your nose contacts your brain's secret responses, bypassing your reasoning self entirely. They also react by passing through the skin itself in minute amounts, acting almost homeopathically to interact with your body chemistry.

Since the dawn of time, the human animal evolved from creatures whose survival depended in part on their sense of smell. Because you are the product of this evolutionary process, you retain this facility. Because it is connected to you on such a primal level, smell reacts without your conscious knowledge or will. It is both a subtle and direct pathway to making changes in both physical health, emotional well-being and higher awareness. Your sense of smell is the sense tied closest to memory. The most casual whiff of certain smells can cause pleasure or relaxation, or wariness and revulsion although you may not be consciously aware that you are smelling anything or what that smell reminds you of.

Your skin also reacts to this molecular cloud. Both a sensory organ and the largest organ of your body, your skin serves a wonderful variety of functions beyond the sense of touch. Being porous, it eliminates toxins along with perspiration. This porosity also allows it to transmit elements into the body on a microscopic level that ever so subtly affect its delicate chemistry.

Your physical body is surrounded by subtle fields of energy that are the manifestation in this universe of your connection to higher states of awareness. These are the physical manifestation of your mental, emotional, spiritual and physical energy levels. These energy fields are also affected by this molecular cloud. By using scented oils, bath crystals, incense and scented smoke to create whatever cloud of fragrance you desire, you can create the type of energy and reaction you want to tune your energies on all levels to a specific purpose.

Essential Oils

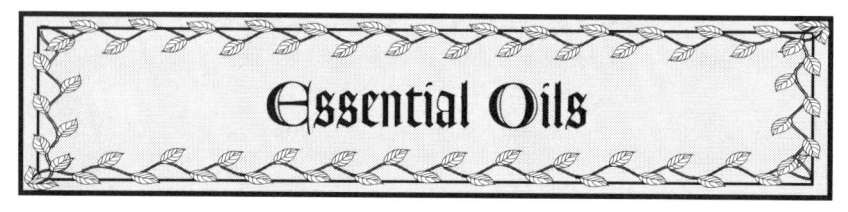

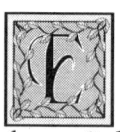

Essential oils are the distilled powers of the plants' potency. Each plant has its own unique fragrance that is as distinct in its identity and energy pattern as the lattice of a crystal. Through their life processes, plants take the energies from the sunlight, moonlight and the earth they are rooted in and transform them into their own life force. This vital essence is stored in their oil glands. Just as no two species of animals are exactly alike, each plant is unique in its identity and in the energy characteristics it creates in its essential oils. Each concentrated essence represents the soul of the plant, the distillation of its very life essence, the carrier of its energy. The life of a plant is intimately connected with the cycles and seasons of the universe. Its life and death are determined by the cycles of the sun and moon. It is integrated in its deepest fibre with the clockwork of the universe. When an oil is taken from the plant, this sensitivity is part of its essence and is carried with the other energies in its makeup. So we say that plants are ruled by certain stars and have the traits of one of the four elements. They exhibit the characteristics embodied by those planets and elements that rule them.

Essential oils can be used in a variety of ways to make this essential energy available. You can release them in smoke by using incense. This will fill an entire room with their fragrance. Continued use of incense in an enclosed space will permeate the curtains and walls with their fragrance so that the room will smell pleasantly even if you do not have the incense burning. If you are sensitive to smoke or wish a lighter fragrance, you may use an infuser in place of incense. This is a small pot usually with a candle flame underneath it. Fill the pot with water and put a few drops of the oil in it. As the candle flame warms the water, the oil's fragrance is released.

You can wear them as perfume oils by putting small amounts of them on the body's pulse points where the skin's warmth will activate their scent and subtle energies. This effect can be increased by putting a few drops in your bath water. While the fragrance fills the space and acts on the subtle senses, the oil itself coats and penetrates the skin acting throughout the body to carry the oil's benefit. Essential oils are extremely concentrated; small amounts of them are very powerful. One drop from the rim of a vial can go a long way and last for hours. It is possible that some concentrated oils can irritate the skin. Before using them in large quantities you should test them individually on the soft skin inside the elbow. Just a touch will do to be sure that they will not irritate your skin.

If you find a fragrance that you wish to have surround you constantly, put a few drops of it on a cotton ball or used dryer sheet when you dry your clothes or linens. This is a wonderful and subtle way to have your bed infused with a restful or dream inducing fragrance while you sleep that will be gently released at every turn of your head on the pillow.

Sometimes wearing essential oils on your skin would not be convenient. Put a drop or two of the oil on a cotton ball and place it in a fabric bag to hang around your neck or put in your pocket. The effect on your body's energies will not be as strong because the oil will not be in contact with the skin, but the fragrance will still act strongly on your subtle senses and act as an enhancement to magical or healing work.

There are an almost limitless variety of essential oils and their combinations to choose from, depending on your intent and purpose. Many of them are listed in the following chart to give you an idea of the range of possibilities for their use. They are listed with their planetary rulership sign and the elements that typify their properties so that you can more easily integrate them in your magickal working.

The Powers of Essential Oils

- ☉ .... Sun
- ☽ .... Moon
- ☿ .... Mercury
- ♀ .... Venus
- ♂ .... Mars
- ♃ .... Jupiter
- ♄ .... Saturn
- ♅ .... Uranus
- ♆ .... Neptune
- ♇ .... Pluto
- ⊕ .... Earth
- † .... Indicates a Fragrance Blend

Essential Oil	♄	Element	Magical	Spiritual
Absinthe †	♂	Fire	Protection - Love Blessing	Psychic Powers
Acacia	☉	Air	Protection	Psychic Powers
Adam & Eve	♀	Water	Love - Happiness	Base Chakra
Allspice	♂	Fire	Money - Luck Healing	Belly Chakra
Almond	♀	Air	Prosperity	Wisdom
Amber	♀	Water	Love Happiness	Strength
Ambergris †	♀	Air	Love	Awakening passion
Anemone	♂	Fire	Health Protection	Energy
Anise	♃	Air	Protection Purification	Harmony Balance
Apple Blossom	♀	Water	Love - Happiness	Uplifting
Apricot	♀	Water	Love Creativity	Mental openness
Aster	♀	Water	Love	Unconditional Love
Azalea	♀	Air	Purification	Clarity Calms
Balsam, Fir	♀	Air	Prosperity	Mental clarity
Banana	♀	Water	Prosperity	Health
Bay	☉	Fire	Protection Purification Healing Attract Women	Calms Psychic Powers
Bayberry	♀	Air	Money - Prosperity	Energy - Clarity
Benzoin	☉	Air	Purification Prosperity	Comforts Calms Balances
Bergamot	☉	Fire	Money	Encouraging Anti-Depressant Balancing
Birch	♀	Water	Protection Purification	Cooling Soothing emotions
Blue Bonnet	♀	Air	Prosperity	Strength Mental Clarity
Camellia	☽	Water	Prosperity	Gentleness
Camphor	☽	Water	Divination	Clarity

14

Essential Oil	☌	Element	Magical	Spiritual
Carnation	☉	Fire	Protection Blessing	Stimulates Strengthens Strength
Cedar	☉	Fire	Money Healing Protection Purification	Calming Comforting Strengthening
Chamomile	☽	Water	Money Love Purification	Calming Relaxing
Cherry	♀	Water	Love	Divination
Cherry Blossom	♀	Water	Peace Harmony Happiness	Balancing
Cinnamon	☉	Fire	Psychic Powers Protection Love - Power	Stimulates creativity Antidepressant
Citronella	☉	Air	Purification	Optimism
Citrus	☉	Air	Psychic Powers Healing	Clarity Mental Focus
Civet +	☉	Fire	Love	Base Chakra
Cloves	♃	Fire	Protection Prosperity Purification Love	Mental powers
Clover	♀	Air	Protection Prosperity Love - Fidelity	Antidepressant
Coconut	☽	Water	Love Courage Protection	Inner peace
Crab Apple	♀	Air	Protection	Uplifting
Cranberry	☉	Fire	Healing Protection Defense	Eases tension Brightens Inspires
Cumin	♂	Fire	Protection Exorcism Love - Fidelity	Dispels negativity
Cyclamen	♀	Water	Fertility - Passion Protection	Heart Chakra
Cypress	♄	Earth	Comfort Longevity Protection	Mental powers
Dove's Blood +	♀	Water	Love Petitions	Magnetic to higher vibrations
Dragon's Blood	♀	Fire	Love Protection Exorcism	Crown Chakra Control of energies
Eucalyptus	☽	Water	Healing Protection Exorcism	Stimulant Heightens Mental Focus

Essential Oil	☿	Element	Magical	Spiritual
Evergreen	☉	Fire	Money Healing Protection Purification	Clarity Calming Comforting Strengthening
Five Finger (Cinquefoil)	♃	Fire	Money Protection	Prophetic Dreams
Frangipani	♀	Water	Magnetizing Attracts opposite sex Love	Stimulates heart and Base Chakra
Frankincense	☉	Fire	Protection, Exorcism Purified Uplifts, Strengthens And Dignifies	Promotes receptivity And Spirituality Aids meditation
Frankincense & Myrrh †	☉ ☽	Fire	Protection Exorcism	Spirituality
Freesia	♀	Air	New beginnings New Awareness	Opening and Stimulating of the heart Chakra
Galangel	♂	Fire	Protection Passion Prosperity	Psychic Powers
Gardenia	☽	Water	Love - Peace	Spirituality Stimulates the heart Chakra
Gardenia Blend †	☽	Water	Love - Peace	Spirituality
Geranium	♀	Water	Love - Fertility Protection	Calming Balancing Antidepressant
Ginger	♂	Fire	Prosperity Love Power Healing	Strengthens Warms the spirit
Ginger Blossom	♂	Fire	Love Passion Healing	Warms the spirit Base Chakra
Ginseng	☉	Fire	Love Beauty/Passion Healing - Vitality	Inner radiance
Grape	☽	Water	Prosperity Fertility	Mental clarity
Grapefruit	☉	Air	Protection Healing	Antidepressant Strengthens spirit & self-esteem
Green Apple	♀	Water	Divination	Psychic insight
Heather	♀	Water	Protection Luck	Optimism Clarity
Heliotrope	☉	Fire	Exorcism Prosperity Invisibility	Soothes nerves Calms Control Anxiety
Hemlock	♄	Water	Power	Astral Projection

Essential Oil	☌	Element	Magical	Spiritual
Hibiscus	♀	Water	Love Passion	Divination Union of upper & lower Chakras
High John the Conqueror	♂	Fire	Prosperity Protection Love	Repels negativity, negative intentions & Adverse conditions
Hollyberry	♂	Fire	Protection Luck Dreams	Openness of Intuition Prophetic Dreams
Honey	☉	Earth	Love Prosperity	Calms Relaxes Balances
Honey Beeswax	☉	Earth	Love Prosperity	Relaxes Balances
Honeysuckle	♃	Earth	Prosperity Protection	Relaxing Soothing, Uplifting Psychic Powers
Hyacinth	♀	Water	Love Happiness Protection	Optimism
Hyssop	♃	Fire	Purification Protection	Mental powers Clarity Creativity
Jasmine	☽	Water	Love - Money Dreams Antidepressant Aphrodisiac	Spiritual love Raises vibrations
Juniper	☉	Fire	Purification Protection Love	Strengthens Antidepressant Centering
Lavender	♀	Air	Love - Peace Purification Protection	Calming Balancing Strengthening Stimulating
Lemon	☽	Water	Purification Love Friendship	Clarity Calming Mental powers
Lemon Grass	♀	Air	Psychic Powers Passion	Tonic Refreshing
Lemon-Lime †	☽	Water	Purification Love Friendship	Clarity Stimulates Antidepressant
Lilac	♀	Water	Exorcism Protection Peace - Harmony	Mind Clearing Aids memory & concentration
Lily of the Valley	♀	Air	Happiness	Mental Powers Optimism
Lime	♀	Water	Friendship Strength	Stimulates Strengthens Antidepressant

17

Essential Oil	☿	Element	Magical	Spiritual
Linden Blossom	♃	Air	Protection Strength Luck	Stimulates Strengthens Antidepressant
Lotus	☽	Water	Protection	Relaxing & cooling
Magnolia	♀	Earth	Love - Fidelity	Purity Clear thinking
Mandrake	☿	Fire	Protection Love - Fertility Prosperity	Control of spiritual energies Power
Marjoram	☿	Air	Protection Love - Happiness Prosperity	Relaxes nervous Tension and Exhaustion
Mimosa	♄	Water	Protection Purification Dreams Love	Soothes worries Lifts spirits
Mint	☿	Air	Passion Protection Travel Exorcism	Refreshing Clarity Increases memory and Concentration
Mistletoe	☉	Air	Protection Exorcism Love - Fertility	Dispels negativity
Mugwort	☿	Earth	Astral Travel Prophetic Dreams	Psychic Powers
Musk	☿	Earth	Enhanced personality Strengthens determination	Strengthens focus
Myrrh	☽	Water	Protection, Exorcism	Spirituality Cools emotions Balances Stimulates brow & crown Chakra
Narcissus	♆	Water	Divination	Strengthens connection with other planes
Nutmeg	♃	Fire	Luck Prosperity Fidelity	Strengthens Calmative Increases dreams
Obeah	♃	Fire	Protection Power	Strengthens Stimulates power
Olibanum	☉	Fire	Protection, Exorcism	Spirituality Aids meditation Antidepressant
Opium	☽	Water	Dreams Sleep Love - Aphrodisiac	Prophetic Dreams
Orange	☉	Fire	Love Prosperity Divination Luck	Relaxing Balancing Stimulating Sensual

Essential Oil	♁	Element	Magical	Spiritual
Orange, Mandarin	☉	Fire	Happiness Joy	Calming Relaxing Antidepressant
Orange, Blossom	☉	Fire	Love Magnetic Attraction Success Compelling persuasion	Calming Relaxing Antidepressant Stimulates belly & heart Chakras
Orchid	♀	Water	Love	Inner beauty & harmony
Orris	♀	Water	Love Protection Divination	Communication with higher beings
Pikaki	♀	Water	Love - Passion	Unconditional Love Fidelity
Papaya	☽	Water	Love Protection	Intuition
Passion Flower	♀	Water	Friendship	Peace
Patchouli	♄	Earth	Prosperity Passion - Fertility	Aphrodisiac
Peach	♀	Water	Love - Fertility Exorcism Wishes - Luck	Dispels negativity Strengthens connections with higher spirits
Pennyroyal	♂	Fire	Strength Protection	Peace
Peony	☉	Fire	Protection Exorcism	Dispels negativity
Peppermint	♀	Fire	Purification Psychic Powers Healing	Antidepressant Mental clarity
Persimmon	♀	Water	Luck Healing	Optimism Clarity of focus
Pine	♂	Fire	Fertility Prosperity Exorcism Protection	Strengthening Cleansing Regenerative
Pineapple	☉	Fire	Luck Prosperity	Energizes Balances
Plumeria	♀	Water	Love	Passion
Poppy	☽	Water	Sleep Love - Fertility Luck Invisibility	Intuition Prophetic dreams
Primrose	♀	Earth	Protection Love	Unconditional love Spirituality
Raspberry	♀	Water	Protection Love	Optimism Brightness & clarity
Redwood	⊕	Earth	Wisdom Connection with higher energies	Balancing & Empowering

Essential Oil		Element	Magical	Spiritual
Rose, Red Rose, White Rose, Wild Rose, Yellow	♀	Water	Love Luck Love Divination Protection Peace	Balancing Strengthen heart Chakra & spirit
Rose Geranium	♀	Water	Protection	Removes sadness and fear
Rosemary	☉	Fire	Protection Love - Passion Mental Powers Purification	Uplifting Mental stimulant Builds strength of character Courage
Rue	♂	Fire	Healing Exorcism Love	Purification Dispelling negativity
Saffron	☉	Fire	Love - Passion Happiness	Psychic Powers
Sage	♃	Air	Wisdom Protection Purification	Cleanses Balances Strengthens
Sandalwood	☽	Water	Protection Exorcism	Spirituality Harmonizing
Sandalwood Parvati +	☽	Water	Wishes Psychic powers	Calming Aphrodisiac
Sassafras	♃	Fire	Prosperity	Strengthens Energizes
Sesame	☉	Fire	Prosperity Passion	Base & heart Chakras
Snowdrops	♀	Air	Rejuvenation Renewal of energies	Spiritual Reawakening
Spanish Moss	♄	Earth	Protection	Dispels negativity
Spearmint	♀	Water	Love Mental Powers	Inner clarity
Spikenard	♀	Water	Fidelity Health	Harmonizing Balancing Stimulates heart Chakra
Strawberry	♀	Water	Love Luck	Joy
Sweet Pea	♀	Water	Love - Friendship Courage Compelling - Drawing Strength	Loyalty Devotion
Sweetgrass	♀	Air	Calling Spirits	Spiritual Attunement
Tangerine	☉	Fire	Protection Defense	Eases tension Soothes Inspires

Essential Oil	☽	Element	Magical	Spiritual
Thyme	♂	Fire	Health Courage Purification Love	Strengthens
Tuberose	☉	Fire	Protection Love Aphrodisiac	Centers emotions Compliments character
Tulip	♀	Earth	Prosperity Love Protection	Awareness of the earth spirit
Van-Van +	♀	Air	Mental powers	Clarity
Vanilla	♀	Water	Passion Mental Powers	Calms Soothes nerves Relaxes
Verbena	♀	Earth	Prosperity Love - Peace Protection Purification	Calms Improves concentration
Vetivert	♀	Earth	Love Luck Prosperity Hex Breaking	Grounding Regenerative Strengthening Aphrodisiac
Violet	♀	Water Luck	Protection Soothes Passion Wishes Reuniting	Stimulates throat chakra Healing
Walnut	☉	Fire	Wishes	Mental Powers
Water Lily	☽	Water	Luck Protection	Psychic Abilities
Wintergreen	☽	Water	Protection Healing Hex Breaking	Aids memory
Wisteria	♆	Water	Protection	Calls aid from higher spiritual forces
Wormwood	♂	Fire	Calling Spirits Protection	Psychic Powers
Ylang-Ylang	♀	Water	Love Peace Calming Tension relieving	Balancing Strengthens spirit Aphrodisiac Magnetic to higher vibrations
Yula	♆	Water	Spiritual & magickal protection	Strengthens connection to higher plane energies
Zula-Zula	♃	Air	Celestial	Magnetic to high vibrations

The Harmonics of Fragrance

Pure essential oils can powerfully affect your senses and energies. When they are combined, they present an almost limitless tapestry of scent and energy. Choose one of these blended fragrances or try mixing one of your own. Go slowly and let each subtle nuance of fragrance play its part in the overall effect.

Apple Spice	The wonderful aroma of apple spice pie baking.
Bay Rum	Bracing clean scent of Victorian after shave.
Blue Sonata	Cool, sweet fragrance reminiscent of starlit nights by a mountain forest lake.
Bouquet, English	Sweet old-fashioned fragrance of an English rose garden.
Bouquet, Floral	Blend of rich sweet flower essences.
Bouquet, Indian	The scent of sandalwood and exotic flowers whispers of faraway places.
Bouquet, Oriental	Exotic and enticing blend of exotic spices.
Bouquet, Spice	Delicious smells of Christmas baking.
Bouquet, Spring	Fresh sweet smell of the first blossoms of the year.
Chocolate	The world's favorite flavor surrounds you with its tantalizing scent.
Country Woods	Comfortable smell of woods and forests.
Flower Garden	Sun warmed medley of spring and summer flowers.
Four-Leaf Clover	Clover and spice for luck and happiness.
Herb Garden	Sharp clean fragrance of green growing herbs.
Herbs & Spices	All the good smells of the herb cabinet are recalled together.
Oriental	Mysterious fragrance inspired by the perfumes of the Far East.
Ouija	Secret aroma recalling ancient temple rites.
Nature	Rich blend evoking the beauty of Mother Earth.
Potpourri	Pleasing fragrance of flowers and herbs adds comfort to any room.
Rainfall	Refreshing scent of rainwater breezes.
Rainforest	Heady scent of ferns and tropical flowers blended with exotic woods.
Summer Garden	Rich green smell of flowers and lush vegetation warmed by the summer sun.
Tutti Frutti	Happy smell of candies and ice cream.
Wildflowers #1	A blend of fragrances from the sunlit fields and meadows.
Wildflowers #2	A blend of fragrances from the shadowy woods and glens.

The Elements of Magick

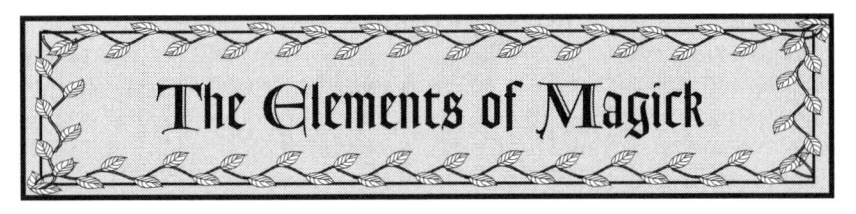

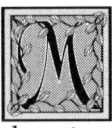

Magick is the art and practice of using energy to influence and alter events on the physical plane. The physical plane is rigid and solid and not easily influenced, but it is interconnected to other planes that are much more flexible and malleable. By changing the energies on those levels, you can change their reflections in this one. Just as you are connected and anchored in this universe by your physical body, you are connected to these other planes with your mental, emotional and spiritual bodies. Each has an existence and awareness unique to it on each of the corresponding planes. Your connection to these other levels of awareness is seen on this plane as the energy shells around your physical body called the Aura or etheric bodies. By working with the energy in these energy bodies you manipulate the energies on other planes that connect to them. This influences the way these other plane energies manifest and, as a result, changes how these energies manifest on this plane. The name for this principle is the "Law of Correspondences". This is the way all sympathetic magick works and it is a very powerful principle.

Because this is a physical universe, nothing can participate in it without a physical vehicle or mechanism that obeys the laws of this universe. Nothing can happen or be experienced without having a physical process involved. This is where the change begins. This is the point of connection and the way you will bring the reality through.

The first step in the magickal process is to work with the energies of your inner universe in order to effect the energies of the greater universes connected to them. Scent, smoke and oiled bath water work on the physical level to bring about the desired change in the energies of your aura bodies. You can use the energy of fire and colored light produced by candles to key into your objective and work with the object of your desire on many levels at once. The most effective way of doing this is to create a physical point of focus. This is a private place that will not be disturbed, preferably in a place where you are not likely to be interrupted. The space does not have to be large, the end of a bookshelf will do. It should be in a place where you can be comfortable, sit with it and use it as a physical point of focus on which to medititate and concentrate the focus of your will upon your desired result.

This space will represent a "mini-Universe", each object in it representing its counterpart in the larger physical world. These objects will all contribute to building a composite of energy that will be as much like the energy pattern of your goal or objective as is possible. Each element will resonate in harmony with the energy level that corresponds to it in your goal or objective. This will draw your goal into reality on this plane. You can call this collection of energies an "essence portrait" because its energies form an energy likeness of your goal or objective that is connected to and will strongly influence the physical plane reality you wish to manifest or change.

Creating a Universe

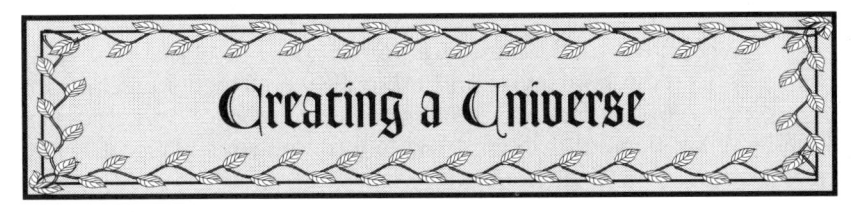

The Essence Portrait

The five elements are one of the most important concepts in magick. It could be said that everything in creation is composed of one or more of these elements in combination. The five elements are symbolic of many of the most basic concepts of our reality. They represent times of life, the levels of awareness, seasons, the winds and the compass points. They also are representative of the states of stages through which pure spiritual energy passes as it manifests in this universe, and correspond to the four planes of existence which make up this particular universe.

Whenever you set a magickal space or do magickal work, invoking the five elements is an important part of setting up the space because by doing that you are constructing a miniature universe that is intimately connected to all the planes and levels of reality. Using specially formulated oils and incense at each of the elemental quarters can enhance both their strength and their presence. You can also work with the elements singly for the purpose of self-development by using them as a focal point of mediation and journey work. If you feel that you need more of a certain quality in your life, working with that element can be very beneficial to helping balance your nature and life. After your initial work with a meditation or drawing ritual, wearing the fragrance on your person can strengthen and enhance your connection with those energies and help bring them into reality in your life and consciousness.

ELEMENT	AIR	FIRE	WATER	EARTH
Direction	East	South	West	North
Spirit	Sylphs	Salamanders	Undines	Gnomes
Archangel	Raphael	Michael	Gabriel	Uriel
Age	Birth	Child	Adult	Old Age
Time	Dawn	Noon	Sunset	Midnight
Season	Spring	Summer	Autumn	Winter
Level of Awareness	Spiritual	Mental	Emotional	Physical

When you build an essence portrait of your object, you must connect it to these four levels and bring all the elements together for your purpose in this physical universe. This is not as complicated as it sounds. What it amounts to is assembling components whose energies closely mirror your goals or objective.

Candles, incense, oils, herbs and stones play an important part in the process of spellwork by making energy patterns on multiple levels. By choosing these components carefully you can put together a working energy model of your objective with your will and desire being the key that turns it on. This "essence portrait" is a combination of images, scents, and objects that carry the closest possible vibration to the feeling of your objective. You are building a focal point for this objective that will be active on many levels at once. It will include incense and scented oil of the appropriate scent, a candle or candles in a color corresponding to the nature and elements of the work, pen, ink and paper or parchment to write out your objective, and, if possible, an image or symbol - whether a photograph, magazine picture and artists rendering - realistic or symbolic - of what you wish to achieve. At times you will also want to include bath crystals, especially when you are doing work on your personal growth and development. Each of these elements plays a singular part in building this essence image by contributing its particular vibrational element to resonate with the higher archetypes and with your inner energies.

Air

Air is the point where all things begin; the place where pure spirit enters this universe. Air represents ideas and concepts and could be described as inspiration before taking action. It represents the Higher Self and the Higher Planes where the essence of all things begins. Air is the Breath of Life symbolized as Dawn or Birth.

Air is identified with the East, the direction of dawn and new beginnings. It is in the east that the first stirrings of the pre-dawn breeze herald the beginning of a new day.

Air elementals are called *Sylphs* and are often pictured as winged sparkling fairies. Birds, angels and other winged creatures of the air have been thought of as divine or heavenly messengers in many cultures - the type of bird specifiying the deity from whom the message came or the nature of its content. It is from this belief that we get the phrase "A little bird told me". On many levels air describes the first stirring of life, the dawn of your idea, the intuition or inspiration, the first step in a process that sets the rest in motion in a particular way.

Incense

Incense represents the element of air. The scent of it will trigger your subtle instinctive senses, and the smoke will interact with your aura to activate changes on all your levels of awareness. It will also interact with the vibrations in the room surrounding you to attune your environment to your purpose. This is an important element in bringing all the elements of your spellwork in tune with each other, with your inner self and with the higher planes of energy to which they are connected. As the scented smoke fills your working space, envision the energy of your magickal purpose drawing around you. See with your mind's eye, the smoke fulfilling its purpose whether to cleanse and banish or charge and attract.

Incense comes in several different forms. One of the most familiar is scented sticks. They are convenient and easy to use. You may place them in a special holder or, if you prefer, you may stick them in a bowl filled with earth or sand to hold them upright while they are burning. In either case, be sure that the ashes are not allowed to fall off onto the table or carpet as this could represent a fire hazard. Another way of using incense is by lighting a self-lighting charcoal block and putting a pinch of the incense powder on it to burn. If you use charcoal blocks, you will need a bowl filled with sand or earth, or, if one is available, a bowl with a screen or wire insert that the block can rest on. Do not use a charcoal block in direct contact with a metal plate or ceramic dish. These blocks are very hot while burning and will burn the surface beneath the container unless they are insulated with sand or earth. You may also use the scented cones with the same precautions.

Fire

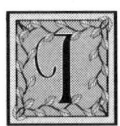

In Fire, the inspiration of Air takes on the first generation of form, becoming action. This is the planning stage of a project where the spiritual impulse of air develops into plans. Fire is the rational mental mind. It is inner fire and vital force whether it is the force that propels an idea into the planning stage or the vital fire which animates a physical body. It is excitement, passion and also good physical health. This is symbolized as Noon or Childhood, and we begin to see the potential of the Infant as self-awareness begins.

Fire elementals are called *Salamanders* and are illustrated as living flames.

The direction of Fire is the South associated with jungles and deserts, the realms where the sun's fierce light is at its most powerful. Its blazing light reveals all parts of the plan, illuminates all phases of a plan and fires the energy it will take to drive the idea towards reality. The ancient legend of the salamander described it as the lizard that could crawl through fire and not be harmed or consumed. Lions are most often associated with fire and sometimes other large cats like cougars and leopards. This comes from their fierce nature and their ancient habit of living in desert regions. In many ancient legends, lions and lion deities are associated with defending the world order against the forces of chaos. This can also be a good analogy for the essence of fire that burns away the fuzziness or disorganization of an inspiration or idea and shapes it into a rational plan of action and energy.

Candles

Candles are an integral part of magickal work. They represent the element of fire, the dynamic principle of inspiration, the spark of life. Colored candles are the power of pure light ray color energy corresponding to the pattern you have set for your goal, powered and driven by the primal fire element. We use candles in magickal workings because the heat and light of the burning wick energize the color of the candle, lending its specific vibrations to the vibrations of the incense and oils already activated. The light of the burning candle unifies all the elements into one focused ray of energy and sets the spell in motion.

Color is a vibration. This means it is a physical manifestation of a specific type of energy. We can experience the pure qualities of specific energies by working with color and light. They correspond to the various frequencies of energy exhibited in the energy centers of your body. These frequencies also correspond to crystals, musical tones, herbs and to the very stars and planets themselves. When fire is the activating agent of this light and color, the power is amplified and released to interact with us on many different levels. When all these elements are combined, the resulting harmonic vibration can be very powerful in acting to change the vibration of the human body, its energy fields and the surrounding environment.

For ordinary spellwork, you will need three candles - the first is the candle that represents the petitioner or the person who is the focus of the spell. If you are working for yourself or for someone whom you know, you may choose a candle that is their favorite color, something that feels harmonious and in tune with the focus of the spellwork. If the subject of the spellwork is not present, you should chose an astrological candle according to their birthday if you know it or corresponding to their most pronounced personality traits if you do not.

The second candle represents the wish or purpose of the work. You will find an extensive list of magickal workings with their candle types and colors at the end of this section. Be sure you hold your purpose clearly and firmly in mind while you dress it.

The third candle is called the Guardian because it joins, steadies and protects the other two. It should be white and as large as or larger than the others because it must burn until they extinguish themselves. It will act as the guard for the others, making sure that the energy remains steady. Should either of the other two be put out accidentally while the work is in progress, you may relight it from the fire of the guardian candle without having to begin the ritual again from scratch.

In The Light

White Light - Power in its purest form. White light generates purity, truth, spiritual strength, clarity of vision and insight. This energy can be used for inner insight and healing, protection, clairvoyance, prophecy and pure focused energy.

Silver Light - Fluidity, psychic gifts, clarity of inner vision, adaptability through change, purifies intention.

Gold Light - Spiritual energy, divine inspiration, divine protection and guidance; attraction and abundance.

Red Light - Attracts and magnetizes passion and sensuality, sex, the opposite sex; strengthens forcefulness, self assertion; strengthens physical vitality.

Pink Light - Attracts affection and romantic love, success, spirituality, assistance of benevolent unseen forces, diplomacy, and femininity.

Orange Light - Solar energy that enhances inner strength and focus. Clarity of mind, self-control, organization, self esteem, friendship and warmth. Aids in attraction and adaptability, vitality, energy.

Yellow Light - Attraction and activity, clarity, concentration and inspiration, agility, cheerfulness, happiness, optimism and luck.

Green Light - Attracts and increases money, abundance, fertility, good fortune, success. Furthers ambition, wealth, finances, healing, health, good crops and harvests.

Blue Light - Truth, wisdom, good health, clarity of expression, wisdom, serenity, peace and harmony in the home, spiritual understanding, calmness and inner peace.

Indigo Light - Force of will, assertion of personal desire and personality from the mental/spiritual plane. Pure intention of command.

Violet Light - Builds and strengthens connection to higher self and higher mind. Dignity, self-assurance, healing of the spirit and inner self, progress, motivation. Enhances psychic abilities and powers.

Brown Light - Earthy and grounding. Sure, steady and stable. Helps with concentration and clarity.

Black Light - Repels and disperses negativity, black magick, sorrow and grief, bad luck.

Rainbow / 7 Colors - For invoking the energies of all the planets together. For full-spectrum healing work where each individual energy will play a part separately as part of the combined whole. For healing and strengthening the Chakras when working with the full energy system rather than a specific center.

The Shape of Your Candles

Most people are familiar with the simple shapes of candles. **Tapers** are the long thin ones of varying length. The length determines how long they will burn. Some are dripless, meaning that the wax entirely consumes itself as the candle burns. Others drip in varying degrees. Be sure that the holder you place them in has a wide enough saucer underneath it in case they drip.

Votive candles are the small chubby ones. They should be burned in a glass or metal holder. You should place the votive holder in a dish or saucer in case the heat of the candle causes the glass to crack and break. This will also protect the surface the votive is sitting on so that it will not become damaged by the heat generated as the candle burns. The wax liquefies quickly after it is lit and the candle will burn for several hours.

Any candle spell can be done with votives or with tapers of varying length, depending on how long you want them to last. There are also other candles available that have different shapes that can contribute to the intent and focus of your spell working. Make your choice according to the meaning of the shape and the color most suited to the focus of your work. These are some popular shapes, but there are many more available at candle and novelty shops. Dress and inscribe a shaped candle just as you would a plain one.

Seven Knot - For wishing. Write the wish along with subject's name and birthday into the wax then, burn one knot per day for 7 days.

Skull - For healing mental and emotional disturbances. Also for developing psychic powers and other plane awareness. For enhancing telepathy. Skull candles will also draw and dissipate nightmares when burned on the bedside table during sleep.

Cat or Snake - For wisdom and to request the aid of a spirit helper or familiar.

Owl - For wisdom and insight.

Dragon - For power and protection.

Male or Female - Write the name and birthday of your subject into the wax. Mark on the back into seven equally spaced sections. Burn the candle each day for a week for the duration of each section.

Unicorn - Connects with magickal and fairy realms. Protects the innocent.

Dolphin - Ocean and water magick. Promotes oneness with nature and harmony with natural forces on all levels and planes.

Moon - Useful when working with lunar magick. Can be used in place of goddess figure in goddess rituals by using shape that corresponds to the lunar aspect of the goddess (Waxing right-handed crescent for Maiden - Full for Mother/Lover - Waning left-handed crescent for Crone/Wise Woman).

Wizard - Use with spirit guide and spirit guardian spells.

Pyramid - The shape of pyramid candles aligns them with higher plane energies and they make excellent vehicles for either banishing or drawing. You can write your complete wish on the bottom as you would do with a piece of parchment as part of the ritual. Then on each side write the word or phrase that would describe how your wish would affect each or your four levels of awareness. Example - If you are working for a better and happier life you would state your complete wish on the bottom of the pyramid. Then on one face you would write "Abundance" and another "Happiness", on the next "Wisdom", and on the last "Good Health". When you dress this candle, bring the oil downward from the tip to the base and picture the energy entering into the candle and grounding into your life. If you are using it to rid yourself of the influence of a person, group, or situation dress the candle from base to tip. Picture the energy flow drawing the negativity out of your life from the base and directing it outward through the tip. As part of your working write the name of the person or group on the bottom along with your complete wish. Then on the sides write the word or phrase desribing how it has affected each of the four levels of your awareness that you wish to banish. Fear, Depression, Poverty, Ill Health, Anger, Pain, Ignorance, Limitation are some good words, but you may have others that more specifically suit your situation.

Preparing Your Candles

Before using candles in your spellwork, you will need to prepare them. This is known as "dressing" the candle.

First, wash them with warm soapy water to remove any grease or dust. Then rinse them in salt water to purify them.

Next anoint them with the appropriate oil. Put a drop of the oil on your finger then, starting at the middle of the candle, rub the oil outward toward the ends until the candle is entirely lightly coated with the oil. Wrap it carefully in plastic wrap or put it in the refrigerator where it will remain clean until you use it.

A Simple Candle Spell

Candle magick can be very simple - as simple as lighting a candle and making a wish. All you need is a candle the color that represents the energy you wish to use and a little oil to dress it with. Colored light energy can be a very powerful meditation tool when you want to reach the pure essence of that vibration. It can also give you a general energy if you do not want to be too specific in your spellwork. If you are working with pure light vibration energy, anoint the candle of your choice with the formula of oil blended to enhance its color energy.

Water

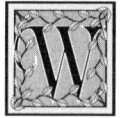

Water is the element of emotions and dreams. It is what connects and communicates between the spiritual higher self and pure reason with our conscious physical world. Water is the point of transformation where inspiration, ideas and energy begin to become concrete, although it has not yet achieved the stability of true form. This is the point of Evening where we can evaluate the results of the day. It also represents Adulthood where the potential of the child is showing results. It is the gate of intuition as it is the point where the fluidity of essential energy encounters the solidity of the physical Universe.

Water represents dreams and visions. This is because it is the point at which what has been pure energy in the first two elements begins to solidify into matter but it is still fluid enough to accommodate the insubstantial nature of Spirit. The West, which is the direction identified with water, is sometimes thought of as the Land of the Dead and the dwelling place of spirits and other world entities.

Water elementals are called Undines and are depicted as mermen and mermaids, but looking much more fishy than human. The vision of the mermaid is very appropriate to this element because it is the mermaid who moves between the dark ocean depths representing the Higher Self and the Subconscious and the bright sunlit world of the sea shore representing conscious, waking reality allowing communication to take place between the two. This is also true of Dolphins and Whales which are the animals associated with this element. They are mammals that live in the ocean and consequenty move from the depths of ocean's darkness to its airy surface like intermediaries between the inner world of consciousness and the outer world of objective observation.

Bath crystals

Bath crystals can be a valuable and powerful part of your ritual process. They help put you in harmony with the flow of the change you are working toward, especially when you are working for personal growth and change. The fragrance of the crystals fills the room triggering your unconscious responses while the essence of the oil penetrates the pores of your skin. A magickal bath also interacts with the energy currents surrounding your body - your aura - to change the vibration of these levels as well. Spellworkings concerning healing, cleansing and banishing are always more effective when accompanied with a magickal bath. But spells of drawing, attracting and enhancing also benefit.

There are three different times during the process of the spellwork that you can take the magickal bath. The first is to bathe before beginning the candle spell. This will attune you to the purpose of the work on many levels and you will be more in harmony with the process as you go on. At other times, such as rituals regarding dream work, you may wish to do the spellwork first and wait until bed time to take the magickal bath so that you will be freshly attuned and in harmony with your purpose while in the dreaming state. If you choose this method, be sure you bless and charge the bath crystals when you are actually doing the candle spell. This will make sure that they are in alignment with your process and that they are tuned in harmony with everything else. The third, is to go through the spellworking and then take the magickal bath to bind and seal your alignment with the changes you are seeking. You will need to use your own judgement about which is most appropriate. Some guidelines are given in the chart of magickal formulas in the next chapter.

Whichever time you select, you should use the same scent as the oil with which you dressed your central candle, the one that represents your goal or purpose. If no specifically prepared bath crystals are available in the formula you need, you can use a few drops of the oil you are using to charge the central candle with in the bath water along with a handful of Epsom salts. Prepare to take as long as you need in your magickal bath. It is part of the meditation process designed to align you with the energies of the changes you want. While in the bath, allow the aroma and feeling of the scent to penetrate your senses. Meditate on the changes you want. Allow the warmth of the water to relax you into a more receptive and magickal state. It might be helpful to light an oiled candle to focus your concentration.

Earth

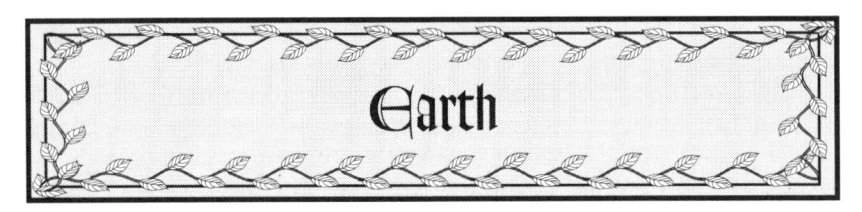

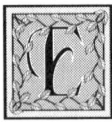

Earth is the last stage in the condensation of matter, where the essence of the other elements comes together into physical reality. Earth is identified with the idea of abundance because it is here that energy is manifested as all possible forms. It is also identified with Midnight, Old Age and Harvest because it represents the culmination of all efforts and energies up to this point. All efforts of shaping energy come to fruition here as the result of the changes brought about through the other three elements. It is the result of the change working in yourself and your life - enhanced awareness, greater knowledge or personal strength, the results of the release from the inhibiting and limiting factors that have controlled your life in this issue.

Earth is associated with the direction North - home of the great ice fields and residence of Winter. It is in the quiet season of winter that the value of the harvest is revealed. The Earth rests and prepares itself for another growing season.

Its elementals are called *gnomes* that appear like fairy tale dwarves who live underground and have charge of all the wealth hidden in the belly of the earth. From olden times the bull or ox has been associated with the element of earth. It was the ox that pulled the plow, turning over the richness of the soil and allowing the abundance of the earth to be sown and harvested. It was also the bull that fertilized the herd to ensure its continuing and the continuing supply of meat and milk.

The element of Earth represents the physical universe reality of your goal or objective. If your work concerns a person, place or object, you should have a picture or representation of that individual, place or thing. If your goal is less concrete such as "Happiness" or "Relaxation", for example, try to find a picture or object that feels the way you imagine your goal would feel if you had it. Whatever you use, the most important part of this component is that it carries both the intellectual intent and the feeling of your objective. It must arouse an inner response in you as well as the mental one of recognition. This is the focal point of your spellworking, the object that will be the focus of manifestation of the energies you want. It is important to have this as concrete as possible.

If you cannot find a picture that feels right, you might want to work with a stone or crystal. By meditating with it you can put the feelings and intentions you have about the issue into it. This will take some concentration and preparation. If you are working with stones, carry the stone you have chosen around with you in your pocket or a bag around your neck, any method that keeps it in contact with you at all times for at least several days before your spellworking. By doing this, it will become charged with your vibration pattern. When you have a chance, at least twice a day, morning and evening, you should take it out, oil it with the oil of your purpose and tell it what you want it to do, and who or what it represents. Work with it between your hands to infuse it with the vibration of your emotions and your goals. After a few days it will take on the pattern of the object you want. When the time comes for your spellworking, anoint the stone or crystal with a little of the oil you used for both the astrological and central candles. Use it as a point of focus during the spellwork just as you would a picture or statue. Remember that if you are doing work to remove and banish energy, it is likely that the stone will retain part of that pattern and it will be necessary to release it when the spellwork is done.

The Energies of Stones

Each type of crystal and stone has its own distinct crystalline formation. When energy of any kind goes through this formation a vibration pattern is emitted. Because the crystal structure of each stone differs from all the others, each vibrational pattern is also unique. It is the nature of stones to focus and enhance specific vibration frequencies. Stones and oils tuned to the stones' vibrational pattern can be very powerful in all types of spiritual and magickal work.

Amber - Amber is not a crystal by the strict definition of the term. It is fossilized tree resin and the process of solidifying and fossilizing have given it the unique properties of a crystalline form. It is distinctly powerful in balancing and regulating the body's energies and will bring strength on all levels, not only physical, but also emotional and mental as well. Its effect is both calmative and energizing and will bring peace strength and lightness of heart. Color range: Pale golden yellow to deep red.

Amethyst - Stimulates the crown chakra to an awareness of higher knowledge and consciousness. Soothes and calms the mundane awareness with the knowledge of a greater perspective. Clarifying to psychic abilities of all kinds. Brings peace and harmony to the spirit because it connects the higher levels of the individual's existence with the physical universe existence. Color range: pale lavender to deep red purple.

Azeztulite - Stimulates the crown chakra and its connection to all higher vibrational planes. Aids in refining the spirit. Provides a tightly focussed channel of energy connected to the angelic realms. Use as an aid to meditation, self-development and personal evolution. Color range: Ice blue to Ice clear.

Charoite - Stimulates the connection between the heart and crown chakras allowing the individual to open to higher conscious awareness. Facilitates mediumship, channelling and psychic abilities and the ability to balance those energies without strain on the physical or mental bodies. Color range: pink-lavender to dark purple.

Citrine - Stimulates the belly chakra and encourages strength of character and identity. Brings about courage and self-assurance and the ability to assert an individual's purpose and personality in the most positive way. Citrine carries gladness to the heart and relief from sorrow and depression. Color range: pale gold through orange to smokey green.

Larimar - Brings peace and healing after work is done. This is healing and rebalancing to all systems providing that the system is at rest. Brings awareness of consciousness in other forms of life and kinship to it. Can aid in finding deep levels of meditation. Color range: Pale to dark blue with red and orange.

Danburite - Stimulates the heart, solar plexus and navel chakras to open and extrovert the individual. This is a powerful mental stimulant that clears away fogginess and brings about mental and emotional openness and steadiness even in the midst of change and external uncertainty. Color range: pale yellow to deep saffron burnt gold.

Emerald - Serves to strengthen and regenerate the heart chakra on all levels. As the energies are used in the process of work or life in general the emerald allows them to be regenerated while keeping the system balanced and refreshed. It is a stone of creativity and abundance because it addresses all levels of generation and renewal. Color range: pale to deep green.

Garnet - Garnet is an earth grounded stone that stimulates the base chakra and strengthens the life force at its entry point. Warms the blood and as a result the heart and mind. Strengthens all levels with basic life fire energy. Warms the heart with passion and helps to focus the power of passion through all levels. Color Range: Rose to red to purple.

Iolite - Stimulates the throat chakra and helps the individual focus on the direction of life or of a specific purpose. Gives focus and personal assertiveness in the ability to pursue a definite course or desire. Color range: clear dark blue.

Lapis Lazuli - Called the Stone of the Seer heightens the ability to develop psychic gifts. Clarifies inner vision, clairvoyance and clairaudience. Strengthens the ability to contact positive spirits. Color range: Indigo blue with gold flakes.

Phenacite - Stimulates the brow and heart chakras to open the individual's capacity to work with each of the chakras separately and together. Balances and harmonizes the aura and allows each of the awareness levels to balance with the others. Facilitates communication with other planes of awareness. Color range: Beige, pink to orange and olive green.

Ruby - Stone of passion and primal fire. Stimulates the base chakra and secondarily the heart chakra on all levels. Encourages openness in the emotions and self-expression when this is due to lack of belief in one's own abilities. Color Range: Rose pink to deep red.

Quartz - Stimulates and harmonizes with all chakras, quartz is the most sympathetic to the human brain wave pattern and as such is an excellent tool to amplify and focus any desired energy on all levels of awareness. Color range: clear.

Rose Quartz - Stimulates the heart and base chakra harmonizing with the energy of love and fidelity. Rose quartz heals the heart chakra by strengthening it and allowing it to reach beyond any negativity that may be affecting it. Supports and energizes any energy system debilitated by injury, illness or emotional stress. Revitalizes the will to live and life force essence. Color range: pink to red.

Sapphire - Stimulates the throat chakra to express the personal will force of the individual. Lends to clear speaking. It is helpful in the development of psychic and magickal abilities in that it allows the wearer to speak and articulate what is perceived as intuition and instinct. Clarifies the will and the expression of its force as desire. Color range: pale to indigo blue.

Seraphinite - Excites and activates the subtle energy system stimulating vitality, energy and warmth on all levels. This enables the individual to reach beyond the temporal physical self and access other levels of power and wisdom. Color range: white.

Sugilite - Stimulates the opening of the crown chakra and alignment of the entire chakra system to attune to this higher vibration. It opens the way for the individual to receive higher knowledge and inspiration. It opens the way to self-knowledge and self-acceptance - a knowledge of oneself as an extension of the greater universe. Color range: violet-pink to purple.

Tanzanite - Stimulates the throat, brow and crown chakras bringing insight and discrimination in all matters. Opens the channels to perception and communication of higher vibrational energies aiding in channelling and psychic abilities. Color range: clear to blue and bluish purple.

Topaz - Stimulates both the brow and solar plexus chakras acting primarily through the mental body. This is the stone of wit and clarity. It brings about brightness of mind and heart and joy founded on the ability to change with agility and purpose. This is sometimes called the Stone of the Dancer because it enables the individual to maintain balance and rhythm through all the changing situations in life due to clarity of mind. Color range: pale to dark yellow gold.

Zincite - Stimulates base and navel chakras to open the way for self assertion and strength of identity which will result in removal and dissolution of energy blockages. Allows a synthesis of personal power, physical vital energy, and creativity on the mental, emotional and spiritual levels. Color range: pale yellow through orange to deep red.

Some of the above stones may appear in other colors. These are the most common.

Spirit

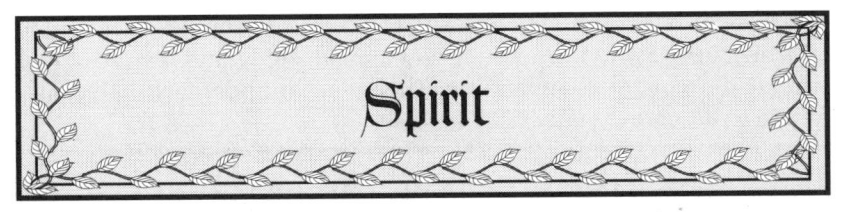

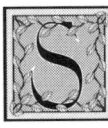

Spirit is the fifth element which is present in all things and binds all things together. It is the true element from which this Universe was created and it could be said that all the others are simply states or conditions in which spirit manifests on this plane.

An important part of your spellwork is your written wish or declaration. This is a critical part of your magickal process because it states exactly what you wish to occur as a result of your work. It is one way in which the element of spirit is present in your elements. Spirit is the unifying factor in all Creation. Your declaration is the unifying factor of your spellwork, the focal point that unifies all the others and moves them to your purpose. The written declaration is very much like an arrow and the magickal work surrounding it is like the bow that shoots the arrow. Both are very important if you wish to bring down your quarry. You should put some time and thought into deciding exactly what you want. Then practice writing it out until you have phrased it in just such a way that it states precisely what you need and want to be the result of your spellwork. This declaration should state your full legal name and your birthday as petitioner. If you are working on behalf of someone else, it should include their full name and birthday if known. It should include the day, date and time you are working. A brief and precise statement of what your purpose is and a final closure such as "Amen" or "So Mote it Be" and your signature.

The date, time and moon phase when you are working
I, (*Your full name*), **born on** (*your Birthday*),
do declare and desire that (*state your wish here*).
So mote it be!

The final writing of the declaration is part of the spellwork itself. To write out your final declaration or petition, you should have a quill or staff pen that you use only for spell work and a piece of parchment. The ink you chose should also be a magickal one chosen to suit the particular purpose you have in mind. When you are done you should fold the paper in thirds long ways like a business letter and in thirds again from side to side so that it makes a closed package. You should be careful to fold the paper away from you if you are banishing and toward you if you are drawing or commanding. Then place it underneath the center candle representing your object or wish.

INK	COLOR	PURPOSE
Attraction	Red-Orange	For drawing to you what you most desire
Blessing	Purple	For drawing an ensuring good energy and protection on whatever you desire
Cleansing & Banishing	Dark Purple	For stating what you wish to be rid of
Dragon's Blood	Red	For any work involving commanding, banishing, exorcising, purging and controlling
Dove's Blood	Rose	For any work involved with wishes and dreams
Fast Luck	Yellow	For changing your luck for the better with speed and ease
Healing	Green	For drawing balancing, healing and harmony on the mental, emotional, spiritual & physical level
Love	Pink	For bringing love and passion into your life
Money	Green	For drawing cash into your life
Reversing	Dark Red	For returning negativity and hex spells back where they came from
Prosperity	Green	For drawing prosperity and abundance on all levels
Protection	Blue-Green	For ensuring the blessing and protection of whatever force or agency is appropriate to the situation
Success	Orange	For drawing success in an endeavor or venture of any type

Tarot

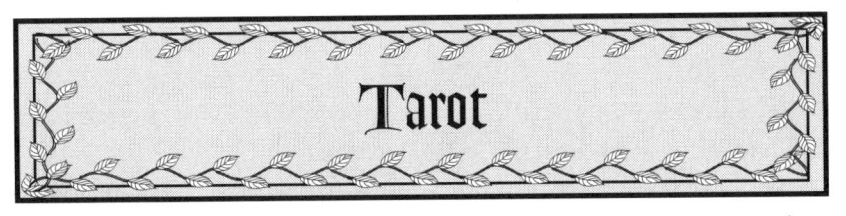

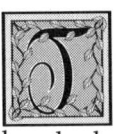

Tarot cards, make excellent tools for your spellworking. Their vivid imagery, subtle coloring and use of powerful symbolism have the power to express their images and deeper meanings on many different levels of awareness at once. There are hundreds of different decks available on the market each with their own distinctive artistic style and particular set of symbolic imagery. It is relatively easy to find just the images that are the most powerful and persuasive for each practitioner's personal taste and senses. Tarot cards also correspond to the planets and the signs of the zodiac. Use the card that most closely illustrates the goal or focus of your work, then enhance its power by using the corresponding scents. Even when you have closed the active phase of your work with the image, the special tarot formula can be worn in a scent bag and carried on your person; or it can permeate your living space in incense or in a warming infuser. Whichever way you prefer or is most convenient, the essence of your work will linger and permeate your environment and interact with you physically, spiritually and psychically on a powerful subconscious level.

Major Arcana Symbology

    0   **The Fool** - ♅ - The Universal Innocent; the Spirit seeking growth and development through experience

    I   **The Magician** - ☿ - Skill, diplomacy, mental activity and agility, dexterity

    II   **The High Priestess** - ☽ - Mistress of secrets yet to be revealed, subconscious, intuition, dreams that reveal answers

    III   **The Empress** - ♀ - Fruitfulness, abundance, beauty, creativity, pleasure, luxury

    IV   **The Emperor** - ♈ - Stability, power, solidity, inner balance, authority and reason

    V   **The Hierophant** - ♉ - Teaching, learning the World's way, Reaching out from the inner world to the outer one, alliances and partnerships

    VI   **The Lovers** - ♊ - Attraction, love, union of opposites

VII   The Chariot -♋- Triumph, the joining of two opposing forces to achieve a goal

VIII   Justice - ♎- Strength and force of law, the power of discrimination and fairness, particularly in legal matters

IX   The Hermit - ♍- Wisdom, guidance from Spirit and higher powers, prudence and care

X   Wheel of Fortune -♃- Destiny, Good fortune, turn of luck for the better

XI   Strength -♌ - Courage, control of one's own nature, taming the wild forces

XII   The Hanged Man -♆- Wisdom, surrender to the will of a higher power or to the hand of fate, surrender to circumstances beyond one's control

XIII   Death -♏- Change, transformation, transmutation, a complete change on all levels preparing for rebirth

XIV   Temperance -♐- Moderation, management, conservation, Nothing dies or is lost; it is transmuted to another form

XV   The Devil -♑- Bondage to the material world, ignorance, limitation, seeing only the surfacing

XVI   The Tower -♂- Destruction, conflict, unforeseen calamities; removal of false preconceptions and attitudes

XVII   The Star - ♒- Insight, hope, inspiration, illumination is available if you open yourself up to it

XVIII   The Moon -♓- Change from within, evolution, spiritual unfolding

XIX   The Sun -☉- Joy, freedom, wealth, good fortune, prosperity work well done

XX   Judgment -♀- Decision that determines a life change, awakening on many levels

XXI   The World -♄- Fulfillment. synthesis, success, rewards gained after labor

Working by the Stars

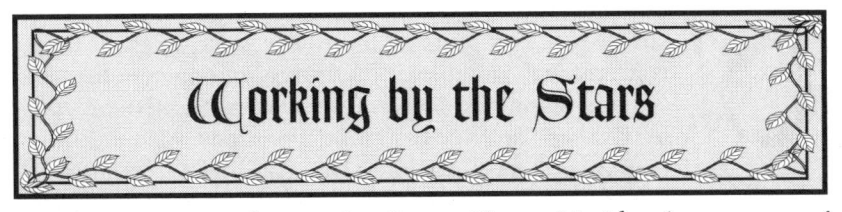

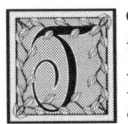

For many thousands of years Humankind has been aware of the forces represented by the planets in our solar system. Each planet represents a unique frequency of energy that is present and active in our lives all the time. The study of the intensity of these energies, their interaction and the effects of this interaction on people and events is called "Astrology". When tuning your magickal work or your essence portrait, you should first decide what planetary rulers your project falls under. Include elements of these planetary forces with your candles and scents to makes your spellworking even more forceful and precise.

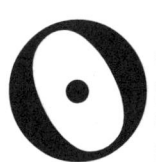

Sun: Rules the general physical health and the vital principle of life. It also rules general prosperity and well being, positions of rank and title such as executive positions and civilian government positions, New ventures, publicity and notoriety, honors and self-esteem, finances, healing.

Moon: Rules women and women's health issues, emotional issues. Travel in safety, protection in all ways, prophetic dreams, reconciliations, all aspects of children.

Mercury: Rules the intellect and learning, and therefore, teaching, printing and publishing. It also rules literature, secretaries, letters, and communications particularly spoken or through the mail. All mental pursuits such as study, concentration and understanding also including psychic development, divination and oracles, opening closed doors and influencing others.

Venus: Rules inner and outer beauty and love. Also the arts, music, painting, sculpture, dancing, poetry. Also cultural activities and places, such as theaters, galleries and museums. Jewelry and beautiful clothing, cosmetics and hairdressers. Peace, happiness, friendships, sexuality, fertility and conception.

Mars: Rules sexual passion, aggression, courage, strength of will and self assurance. Also rules all things concerning the military including people, operations, arms, armaments and explosives (except fireworks that are ruled by Uranus), and honors and decorations. Also machines, engines and mechanics and the working of iron and steel.

Jupiter: Rules judges, administrators, and theologians. Also financial dealings, the stock market and financial prosperity and well-being. Peace of mind due to good financial and material security. Attracts money and material things. Friendships and the good life. Jupiter rules the seeking and granting of favors.

Saturn: Rules land, mines and real estate. Also old people, antiques, junk and junk dealers. Building procedures have to do with the earth such as bricklaying, stone masonry, plumbing and the pouring of concrete. Also pottery. Influences others, business and financial relationships. Its forces deal with discipline and the teaching of life's lessons. Its influence is controlling, binding, limiting and guarding. Develops mediumship and channelling.

Uranus: Rules abrupt and unexpected changes. Metaphysics, radio and satellite communications, air travel, electricity and new inventions. Also clairvoyance, telepathy and psychic abilities in general. The influences of Uranus have to do with love of freedom and independence. It is the motivating force behind a wandering nature.

Neptune: Rules liquids of all kinds, perfumes, mind altering and hallucinogenic drugs. Shipping and ocean voyages. Neptune's influence is seen most strongly regarding inner vision and perception, particularly the vision that tears down the old life to make way for the new, the fruit of the higher vision. It is because of this that Neptune is often thought of as the bringer of chaos, confusion and revolution.

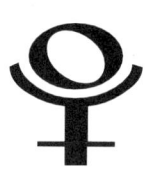

Pluto: Rules transformations, transfigurations and metamorphosis. These can be in the physical world concerning chemistry and alchemy, toxic or lethal drugs, or any kind of gas and vapor. It can also refer to astral travel and the spiritual world in general and materializations in particular.

Planetary Attributes Chart

Planet	Day	Color	Metal	Stone	Chakra	Zodiac
Sun ☉	Sunday	Orange	Gold	Carnelian Citrine	Belly	Leo ♌
Moon ☽	Monday	White	Silver	Moonstone Pearl	Crown	Cancer ♋
Mars ♂	Tuesday	Red	Iron	Bloodstone	Base	Aries ♈
Mercury ☿	Wednesday	Yellow	Quicksilver Brass	Topaz	Solar Plexus	Gemini ♊ Virgo ♍
Jupiter ♃	Thursday	Purple	Tin	Amethyst	Brow	Sagittarius ♐
Venus ♀	Friday	Green Rose	Copper	Emerald Rose Quartz	Heart	Taurus ♉ Libra ♎
Saturn ♄	Saturday	Indigo	Lead	Sapphire	Throat	Capricorn ♑
Uranus ♅	N/A	Changeable	Uranium Aluminum	Opal	---	Aquarius ♒
Neptune ♆	N/A	Turquoise	Platinum	Aquamarine	---	Pisces ♓
Pluto ♇	N/A	Black	N/A	N/A	---	Scorpio ♏

Astrological Candles & Oils

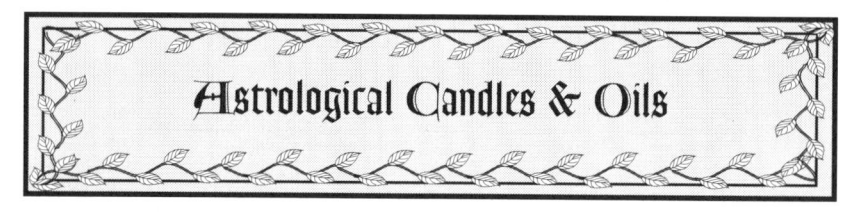

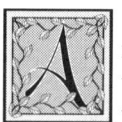

Astrological oils are used to dress the central candle representing the subject of your candle spell. They can also be very potent in enhancing your own work with your astrological nature. Oils make the essence portrait much richer and deeper when working with a person who is not present. If you do not know your subject's birthday, choose a white candle. Then, when you have washed the candle and dressed it with the appropriate astrological oil, write the person's full name into the wax using any sharp point such as a darning needle or pen point.

Aries - (March 21-April 19) - Those born in the Sign of the Ram are independent and active, forceful, dynamic, brave and self-assured. They love challenges and are born pioneers. Element: Fire, Ruler: Mars, Color: Red, Stone: Ruby and Bloodstone

Taurus - (April 20-May 21) - Those born in the sign of the Bull are loyal and generous. They love security and appreciate the good things in life and are not afraid of working to get them. They are gracious and romantic. Element: Earth, Ruler: Venus, Color: Green, Stone: Emerald

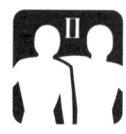

Gemini - (May 22 -June 21) - Those born in the Sign of the Twins are witty and talkative. They are said to have a dual nature that can do several tasks at once. They diversify and change. Element: Air, Ruler: Mercury, Color: Yellow, Stone: Topaz

Cancer - (June 22 -July 22) - Those born in the Sign of the Crab can be shy and sensitive. They are natural nurturers and teachers. They are great lovers of hearth and home and prize tradition and heritage. Element: Water, Ruler: Moon, Color: Silvery Pastels, Stone: Moonstone & Pearl

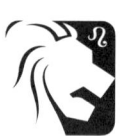

Leo - (July 23 -August 23) - Those born under the Sign of the Lion are theatrical and outgoing, proud of their achievements, chivalrous and noble. They are great lovers of display and pleasure. Element: Fire, Ruler: The Sun, Color: Gold or Orange, Stone: Carnelian

Virgo - (August 24-September 23) - Those born under the Sign of the Maiden are analytical and careful, organized and efficient. Their standards are high both for themselves and others. They are compassionate and respond to those in need. Element: Earth, Ruler: Mercury, Color: Blue and Gray, Stones: Jacinth

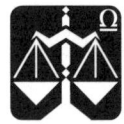

Libra - (September 24-October 23) - Those born in the Sign of the Balance are peace loving, just and eloquent. But their search for balancing everything sometimes makes them seem indecisive. Element: Air, Ruler: Venus, Color: Rose and Blue. Stones: Rose Quartz and Chrysocholla

Scorpio - (October 24-November 22) - Those born in the Sign of the Scorpion are passionate and energetic. They are complex, contradictory and many layered. Sometimes difficult to know, they are loyal and warm to those they love. Element: Water, Ruler: Pluto, Color: Red and Black, Stones: Garnets

Sagittarius - (November 23-December 21) - Those born under the Sign of the Archer are forceful and dynamic, fun loving and optimistic. They are sometimes restless and often plain spoken. Element: Fire, Ruler: Jupiter, Color: Purple and Dark Blue, Stones: Amethyst and Sapphire

Capricorn - (December 22-January 20) - Those born under the Sign of the Sea Goat are serious and single minded. They are conscientious and determined in their pursuit of their goals. Element: Earth, Ruler: Saturn, Color: Dark Blues and Browns, Stones: Amber and Smoky Quartz

Aquarius- (January 21-February 19) - Those born under the Sign of the Water Carrier are idealists and dreamers. They have calm pleasing and agreeable temperaments. They have a natural sense of justice and fairness. Element: Air, Ruler: Uranus, Color: Electric Blue, Stone: Sapphire

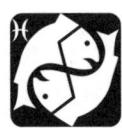

Pisces - (February 20-March 20) - Those born in the Sign of the Fishes are Imaginative, intuitive, introspective and romantic. Pisceans are quiet and excellent keepers of secrets. Element: Water, Ruler: Neptune, Color: Green and Greenish Blue, Stone: Quartz, Opal andAquamarine

Timing Your Work by the Planets

You can make further use of these forces by choosing days and times for your work ruled by the planets most favorable to your purpose. By "ruled" we mean that the desired planet has its strongest influence at this time. Call your local weather bureau or look in the newspaper for the exact time of sunset or use an almanac. The time from sunrise to sunset is precisely 12 hours only on the Equinoxes. There are two ways of getting around this and both methods are equally valid. You may count 60 minute hours beginning from the time of sunrise or sunset until the time your magickal work is done, or you may calculate the number of minutes between sunrise and sunset and divide by twelve, that will give you "hours" either longer or shorter than the standard 60 minutes. Remember that Sunset is considered to begin the first hour of the day. This may take a little getting used to. For instance, Sunday is actually considered to begin at sunset on Saturday. Monday begins at sunset on Sunday, etcetera.

Planetary Hour Charts

Hrs after Sunset	Sun	Mon	Tue	Wed	Thu	Fri	Sat
1st	☉	☽	♂	☿	♃	♀	♄
2nd	♀	♄	☉	☽	♂	☿	♃
3rd	☿	♃	♀	♄	☉	☽	♂
4th	☽	♂	☿	♃	♀	♄	☉
5th	♄	☉	☽	♂	☿	♃	♀
6th	♃	♀	♄	☉	☽	♂	☿
7th	♂	☿	♃	♀	♄	☉	☽
8th	☉	☽	♂	☿	♃	♀	♄
9th	♀	♄	☉	☽	♂	☿	♃
10th	☿	♃	♀	♄	☉	☽	♀
11th	☽	♂	☿	♃	♀	♄	☉
12th	♄	☉	☽	♂	☿	♃	♀

Hrs after Sunrise	Sun	Mon	Tue	Wed	Thu	Fri	Sat
1st	♃	♀	♄	☉	☽	♂	☿
2nd	♂	☿	♃	♂	♄	☉	☽
3rd	☉	☽	♂	☿	♃	♀	♄
4th	♀	♄	☉	☽	♂	☿	♃
5th	☿	♃	♀	♄	☉	☽	♂
6th	☽	♂	☿	♃	♀	♄	☉
7th	♄	☉	☽	♂	☿	♃	♀
8th	♃	♀	♄	☉	☽	♂	☿
9th	♂	☿	♃	♀	♄	☉	☽
10th	☉	☽	♂	☿	♃	♀	♄
11th	♀	♄	☉	☽	♂	☿	♃
12th	☿	♃	♀	♄	☉	☽	♀

The Moon's Influence

The Moon's influence is very powerful. Its phases pull the tides of all of Earth's oceans and, since physical bodies are composed mostly of water, its influence is felt in our internal tides as well. The growth of plants, the reproductive and mating cycles of animals, the migration cycles of many types of creatures are directly tied to the Moon's subtle but powerful pull. The Moon's phases also influence the magickal work that you do. Tuning your work with the phases of the Moon makes use of these powerful forces and will greatly increase the effectiveness and quality of your magick. Using the scents that correspond to these phases enhances the connection to these influences, binding them closer to the focus of your work and maintaining this influence even after the actual time of the phase is past.

The Moon's cycle is 29 days long. It has four distinct phases. Again your almanac can help you find the most productive time for your working.

Waxing Moon - Beginning with a silver thread, the visible face of the Moon grows steadily larger toward full. This is the time to make preparation, bless seeds and make wishes. This is the time of germination and emergence.

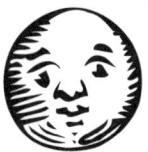

Full Moon - The three days when the Moon is completely full and round are good for celebrating fullness and completion of any project. A good time for social gatherings. Work for any project that needs growth to come to fruition such as love, fertility, and financial ventures.

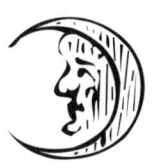

Waning Moon - Work at this time for anything that needs to be removed from your life or anything that you wish to terminate or destroy. This is the time to weed the garden so that the weeds do not grow back. Harvest crops at this time that you intend to plow under or cut your hair if you wish it to remain short.

New Moon - The three days when the moon is fully dark are a time to plan for future work. This phase works well when generating chaos and disintegration, confusion, and downfall, or reversing spells that others have worked. Banish energy in any form to rid yourself of it at the source.

Your magickal wish spell

Now that you have gone over all the elements of your spellwork individually, we'll go over them altogether. When you are putting together your spells you might want to use these pages as a check list to be sure you have not forgotten anything before you begin.

1. **Air** - Incense with a scent corresponding to the purpose of your spell. Holder for stick incense or bowl of sand for charcoal and powdered incense

2. **Fire** - Three candles
    Astrologically oriented for you or the person for whom you are doing the spell.
    Colored candle representing the purpose of the spell
    White guardian candle as large or larger than the other two
   Holders for candles
   Matches or lighter

3. **Water** - Blessing oil for blessing your table surface.
   Oil for dressing the candle's Astrological and Magickal Purpose
   Bath crystals or oil

4. **Earth** - Picture, Image or Tarot card.
   If the picture is one that you wish to keep it would be wise to get a copy of it made, a color xerox will be fine. The picture or stone will become part of the spellworking and should not be returned to regular use. If you cannot get a copy of your chosen tarot card, it can be blessed and cleansed with salt and sage after the spellworking is completed. If you are using a stone or crystal, have it charged before you begin the spell.

5. **Spirit** - Have the text of your wish or declaration prepared before you begin the spell.
   Quill or staff pen
   Magickal or colored ink corresponding to purpose of spellwork
   Parchment or clean white typing paper

6. **Time for working** - Moon phase & planetary hour

7. A small box or tray to put your assembled articles in so that they will be convenient and contained.

8. Choose a private place for your spellwork where your candles will not be a fire hazard and where they will not be disturbed or accidentally extinguished. A wooden surface that can be easily cleaned is best but any firm flat surface will do.

Begin by making sure your chosen space is clean and free from any fire hazards. Dust and wash your table top, then rinse it with sea water or a mixture of salt and water. Then, put a drop or two of the Blessing Oil on your fingertip and draw a line clockwise around the surface's edge.

When your surface is clean and blessed you may begin placing your Spellworkings. First, place the candle signifying the purpose of your work in the center with the candle signifying the subject of the work to its right and the Guardian candle to its left.

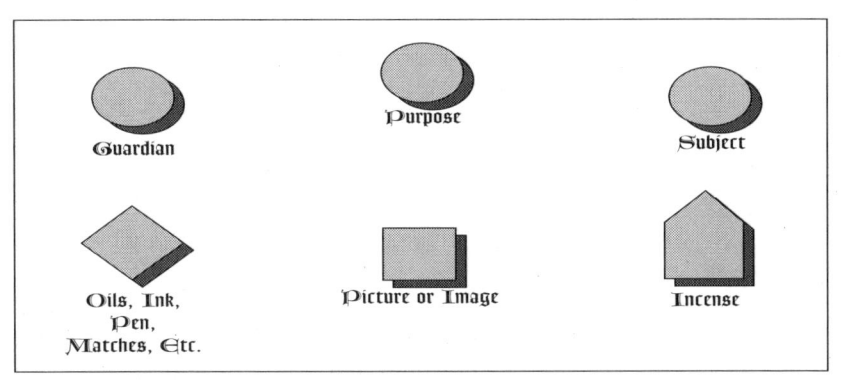

```
     Guardian          Purpose           Subject


  Oils, Ink,        Picture or Image     Incense
    Pen,
  Matches, Etc.
```

Place the oils and incense as is shown above, close enough for easy reach but not so close that you will knock them over in the process of your spell work. Sit down in front of your table and take a deep breath. Relax and allow the stress and tensions of the day to recede. Now is your private time for your magick. Breathe deeply and slowly and allow yourself to become focused on the objects before you. When you feel relaxed and focused it is time to proceed.

Beginning with the center candle, take the appropriate oil and dress each of the candles. On the center one briefly inscribe the purpose for which you are working the date and phase of the moon. On the Subject candle inscribe the name and birthday of the person for whom you are working. On the guardian candle inscribe the name of your guardian spirit or angel if you know it, if not, leave it blank. As you inscribe and oil each one speak your wishes and purpose for it aloud. This is very important to clarifying and manifesting your wish in the physical universe. When your candles are inscribed and dressed, light the center one, then the Subject, then the Guardian.

When you are sure they are burning well, light the incense signifying the purpose of your spell from the central candle and place it in its holder. Make sure there is enough to make a smoke you can see. Inhale this smoke deeply. Make sure it surrounds you and permeates the space you are working in. Take the incense stick and pass it around your body and under your arms and legs. Allow the smoke from the incense to charge and cleanse your aura, your spiritual and physical energy fields, to conform to your purpose.

Now, open the ink and take out the pen and parchment. Transcribe the declaration you have written out onto the parchment. Be sure you include your name, your birthday and the date and time you are working. It should look something like the model declaration shown in the section on magickal inks. When you have finished writing it, hold it up and read it aloud. Make sure you speak clearly and distinctly. Remember, you are setting a process in motion by this act and you want to do it firmly and clearly. Then, fold it carefully in thirds the long way first making sure that if you wish to draw something to you, you fold the edge toward you. If you wish to banish something, you fold with the edge going away from you. Now turn it and fold it in thirds down its length folding either toward or away as before so that the paper makes an enclosed package. Place the folded declaration beneath the central candle. Take your photograph, picture, tarot card or other image and place it in front of the central candle. Make sure to place it so that you can see it easily as you sit in meditation.

Now that the physical part of your spell is set up, you can begin your inner magick. Sit comfortably in front of your spellworking. Allow yourself to relax and become aware of the flickering light of the candles, the scent of the incense, the sensations in your body. Just sit quietly for a moment until you are comfortable and relaxed. Now let your mind focus on the picture or image that you have chosen to represent your goal or object. As your eyes focus on it, hold it in your mind as well. Imagine that you surround the image, that it is inside you and a part of you. Experience its *reality*. Know that whatever you intend has force and power, has reality. See this reality in your mind. Know that it exists and will manifest itself in your life and awareness. Know that your objective is yours; it belongs to you and is part of you. Sit for a while and allow the knowledge of this reality to become a comfortable part of your awareness. Remain sitting here until the incense has burned itself out. If you feel comfortable with your reality then you may depart. If you would like more time to meditate on the reality of your image, take as long as you like. Light more incense if you would like to and continue with your meditation until you feel comfortable.

When you are done you should leave all your candles burning until they burn themselves out. The cycle of energy you have initiated must be allowed to complete its task. If your spellworking is intended to take more than one day, you should repeat your meditation each day at the same time. The guardian candle should burn longer than the others. If it burns quickly and appears that it will not last long enough, get another white candle and light it from the flame of the first one. As long as the guard candle is burning, should either of the others accidentally be blown out, you may relight them from the guardian candle without having to begin the spellworking all over again.

After all the candles have burned themselves out, place anything that remains in a paper bag - any wax drippings, incense ash, the declaration and the picture or image you used. If your spellworking was intended as a blessing or drawing, you should keep these remaining elements of your spellworking. You may bury them in your yard if you have one or keep them in a small container in your dresser or closet if you wish. If your spellworking was one of banishing and reversing, put all the remnants of the spell in a paper bag and carry them away from your house or property. Dispose of them appropriately and return to your house by a different way than the way you came. You should also remember that in disposing of these negative elements you must be willing personally to release the negativity they represent. It will do you no good to go through an entire spellworking to banish a harmful person or situation from your life if you continue to recreate it in your thoughts and emotions. You must be ready to let the situation or individual go. Release it as you do the remnants of your spellworking, and, when you return home, know that you have started a new day in your life that is positive and strong. Your spellworking has planted the seeds of new beginnings, now you must nurture and cultivate what springs from them.

It is important at this time to remember that your objective will come about in a completely natural way. Each universe must operate by its own natural laws. Nothing can exist or happen in any universe that is in any way contrary to the laws that govern it. Although we have seen countless movies where the results of a magickal spell pop out of the air with a bang and a flash of green smoke, it never really happens like that in real life. **But it will happen.**

Know that what you intend will come about within the laws of nature. Do not worry about it. Magick reveals and manifests itself over time in ways that are consistent with this universe. This can be remarkably subtle and you may not notice your results at first. It can be interesting to keep a journal of your spellworking. Sometimes you may not even be aware of a change occurring until you look back on things and see how they have changed.

Magickal Blends

☉. Full Moon   ☽. Waning Moon   ●. New Moon   ☾. Waxing Moon
☉. Sun   ☽. Moon   ☿ ... Mercury ♀.. Venus
♂. Mars   ♃.. Jupiter   ♄ ...Saturn   ♆.. Neptune
♅.. Uranus   ♇.. Pluto

Formula	⚗ ☽ Purpose	Candle Color	Candle Type

Abracadabra ♀ ☾   Orange   Taper/Votive
Spell to increase the force of your magickal work.

Abramelin ☿ ☾   Yellow   Taper/Votive
Kabalistic drawing & opening formula.

Abundance ♀♃ ●   Green   Taper/Votive
To draw plenty & richness of all sorts.

All Purpose
Select the planetary influence and color taper or votive candle most appropriate to your purpose or with white candle at full moon for general power essence. Charge to assist and enhance your magickal purpose.

Alpha ☿☽ ☾   Blue   Taper/Votive
To encourage a meditative, creative and powerful state of mind

Amiability ♃♀ ●   Gold   Taper/Votive
To draw friendship, good feeling & fellowship

Anti-Insomnia ☽ ☽   Blue   Taper/Votive
Prepare a scent bag or sachet pillow during the waning moon. Use with candle as needed.

Anointing   ☉
Consecrate this oil to the desired deity or charge it to the desired purpose at the full of the moon. Use when needed.

Anti-Depression ☉ ●   Orange   Taper/Votive
To raise the spirits & clear the mind.

Anti-Nightmares ☽ ●   Orange   Taper/Votive
Prepare a scent bag or sachet pillow during the full moon. Use with candle as needed to banish night terrors. Bath crystals may be used before retiring.

Anti-Poltergeist ♀ ☽   Purple   Taper/Votive
Spell to banish a noisy, disruptive entity and/or energies.

Formula ☙ ☽ Purpose	Candle Color	Candle Type

Astral Travel ♀ ☾   Blue   Taper/Votive
Spell to safely assist the spirit in letting go of the body to fly free.

Attract a Friend ♃ ☉   Gold   Taper/Votive
Spell to attract companionship.

Attract a Husband ♀ ☉   Green   Taper/Votive/Male
Spell to attract a male life mate.

Attract a Lover ♂ ☉   Pink   Taper/Votive/Male/Female
Spell to attract passion and romance.

Attract a Soul Mate ♀ ☉   Green   Taper/Votive/Male/Female
Spell to attract a spiritual mate and companion.

Attract a Wife ♀ ☉   Green   Taper/Votive/Female
Spell to attract a female life mate.

Attract Business ♄ ☉   Purple   Taper/Votive
Spell to attract commercial opportunities.

Attract Customers ♃☉ ☉   Yellow   Taper/Votive
Spell to attract paying customers to the place of business.

Attract Sales ♃ ☉   Green   Taper/Votive
Spell to move merchandise for cash.

Attraction ♂☉ ☉   Red/Orange/Cranberry   Power 16"
Spell to increase your ability to draw to you what you need and want. Use with bath crystals & scent bag to amplify & bind effect.

Aura Cleanse ♄ ☽   Rainbow   Taper/Votive
Ritual to remove negative vibrations and blockages from the body's energy fields.

Avert Evil Eye ♂ ☉   Red/Black   Taper/Votive
Spell to turn away negative intentions and ill-wishing.

Balancing ☉ ☾   Brown   Taper/Votive
Ritual to bring the body/spirit's energies into harmony with each other and their surroundings.

Banish & Cleanse ♄ ☉   Black/White   Power 16"
                               White/Purple   Taper/Votive
Spell to use before blessing a space, object or person to be certain no negativity remains.

Banish Evil Spirits ♀ ☉   Black   Taper/Votive
Spell to banish negative, harmful entities and energies.

Banish Ghosts ♀ ☉   Black   Taper/Votive
Spell to banish spirits of the dead who are troubling the living.

Formula	☿ ☽ Purpose	Candle Color	Candle Type
Be Faithful	♀ ☾	Pink	Taper/Votive
	Binding spell to keep a lover true.		
Beauty	♀ ☽	Pink	Taper/Votive
	Spell to reveal your own inner beauty, harmony & radiance.		
Become Invisible	☿ 🌍	Yellow	Taper/Votive
	Spell to go about your activities and remain unseen and unnoticed.		
Bend Over	♂ ☾	Red	Taper/Votive/Male/Female
	Controlling & dominating the object of your desires.		
Beta	☉ ☾	Red	Taper/Votive
	Ritual to enhance conscious awareness, focus and clarity on a daily mundane level.		
Binding	♄ ☾	Red	Taper/Votive
	To seal and secure the results of spellwork.		
Bleeding Heart	☉ ☾	Pink/Green	Taper
	Ritual to heal a broken heart. Use with bath crystals & scent bag.		
Bring Back Friend	♃ ☾	Yellow	Taper/Votive/Male/Female
	Spell to restore companionship.		
Bring Back Lost Love	☽♀ ☾	Pink	Taper/Votive/Male/Female
	Spell to restore a loving relationship.		
Centering	☉ ☽	White	Taper/Votive
	To bring you back to your own inner center of light prepare scent bag at full of moon to wear when needed. Use with bath crystals to purify & center aura.		
Ceridwen's Cauldron	☿ ☾	Rainbow	Taper/Votive/7 Knot
	Spell to attract needed knowledge & enlightenment.		
Chakra Showers	☉ ☾	Rainbow	Power 16" or 7-Day
	Ritual to clarify & strengthen the energy centers of the body using scent bag and bath crystals.		
Changes	♅♆ ☽ ☉ ☾	Black White	Taper/Votive
	Spell work to be done twice in one moon cycle during the waning moon to remove old & outworn elements of your life, then again in the waxing phase to bring in the new & beneficial elements using bath crystals and scent bag to reinforce and bind.		

Formula ☿ ☽ Purpose	Candle Color	Candle Type

Channelling ♄ ☾   Indigo   Taper/Votive/Skull
Ritual to open your inner senses and channels to allow beneficial entities to speak through you.

Chastity ♀♄ ☽   Black   Taper/Votive
Spell to insure sexual purity.

Clarity of Mind ☿ ☾   Yellow   Taper/Votive/Skull
Spell to dispel fogginess and increase mental focus.

Cleansing ♄ ☽   Black/White/Purple   Power 16"
Ritual to rid a place or person of all negativity and blocked energy regardless of the source.

Clear Bad Vibrations ♄ ☽   Black   Taper/Votive
Ritual to rid a place or person of all negativity and blocked energy regardless of the source.

Coin & Cash ♃ ☾   Green   Taper/Votive
Spell to bring cash money to you.

Come & See Me ♂ ☾   Red   Taper/Votive/Male/Female
Spell to draw one to you that you would like to see.

Commitment ♂ ☾   Pink   Taper/Votive
Spell to pledge commitment to a relationship, ideal or project.

Communication ☿ ☾   Yellow   Taper/Votive
Spell to clarify and moderate communications between two or more parties.

Compassion ☿ ☽   Pink   Taper/Votive
Spell to send love & compassion to one who needs these healing energies.

Concentration ☿ ☾   Yellow   Taper/Votive
Spell to increase your clarity of focus.

Confidence ☉ ☾   Orange   Taper/Votive
Spell to find your inner self-confidence, self-assurance & self-esteem. Should be used with bath crystals & scent bag.

Confusion ♆ ☽   Black   Taper/Votive
Confound & confuse those who send negativity to harm you.

Cosmic ☿ ☾   Silver   Taper/Votive
Ritual to expand the horizons of your spirit.

Cosmic Consciousness ☿ ☾   Silver   Taper/Votive
Ritual to expand your inner vision of the infinite universe and your place in it.

Formula	☌ ☽	Candle Color	Candle Type
Purpose			

Courage ♂ ☾ Red Taper/Votive/Dragon
Spell to find you inner strength & courage. Should be used with bath crystals & scent bag.

Court ♃ ☾ Purple Taper/Votive
Spell to insure a fair and impartial hearing.

Cupid's Arrow ♀ ☾ Pink Taper/Votive/Male/Female
Spell to draw love from someone you desire.

Desire ♀ ☉ Pink Taper/Votive
Red Male/Female
Spell to awaken desire in someone you love.

Develop Psychic & Mystic gifts ♀ ☾ Orange Taper/Skull
Ritual to increase and deepen your psychic and mystical powers. Use with scent bag and bath crystals.

Devotion ♀ ☾ Pink Taper/Votive/Male/Female
Spell to draw the devotion of a loved one. Use with scent bag and bath crystals.

Divination ♀ ☽ Yellow Taper/Votive/Skull
Ritual to accompany divination process to increase accuracy and perception. Use bath crystals prior to the divination.

Domination ♂ ☉ Red Taper/Votive
Spell for controlling & dominating the object of your desires.

Dove's Blood ♀ Pink Taper/Votive
Spell for making wishes & petitions. Use with bath crystals & scent bag.

Dragon Protection ♂ ☽ Red Taper/Votive
Dragon
Spell to draw the dragon power of the earth to act in you protection and defense. Use with bath crystals & scent bag.

Dragon's Blood ♂ ☽ Red Taper/Votive
Spell used to drive away negative energy of any sorts, purge a space or object and bind it to your will.

Dream ☽ ☾ Silver Taper/Votive/Skull
Spell for use with bath crystals for prophetic or divinatory dreaming. Use with bath crystals & scent bag

Formula ⚯ ☽ Purpose	Candle Color	Candle Type

Dream Come True ☿ ☾   Gold   Taper/Votive/7-Knot
Write your special wish on the candle before you anoint it with the oil.

Elf Vision ☽ 🌑   Silver   Taper/Votive
Spell to see the magickal world of the fairy people. Use with bath crystals & scent bag

Employment ☉ ☾   Orange   Taper/Votive
Spell to find a good job. Use with bath crystals & scent bag.

Empower ☉♂ ☾   Gold   Taper/Votive
Spell to find and access your true source of personal power.

Enchantment ♆ ☾   Turquoise   Taper/Votive
Spell to cause others to see things as you wish them to: an illusion spell.

Enchantment Men ♆ ☾   Turquoise   Taper/Votive/Male
Spell to make men look different than they truly are.

Enchantment Women ♆ ☾   Turquoise   Taper/Votive/Female
Spell to make women look different than they truly are.

Enchantment People ♆ ☾   Turquoise Taper/Votive/Male/Female
Spell to make people look different than they truly are.

Enchantment Things ♆ ☾   Turquoise   Taper/Votive
Spell to make things look different than they truly are.

Endurance ♂☉ ☾   Orange   Taper/Votive
Spell to increase your strength and endurance both emotionally & physically.

Energy Giving ☉♂ 🌑   Red   Taper/Votive
Spell to enable you to draw extra energy & life force. Use with bath crystals & scent bag.

Enhance Personality ☉ ☾   Gold   Taper/Votive
Spell to bring out, focus & amplify your best qualities. Use with bath crystals & scent bag.

Enhancement ☉ ☾   Gold   Taper/Votive
Spell to focus and amplify energy use with bath crystals & scent bag.

Environment ☉ ☾   White   Taper/Votive
Spell to assist in controlling your environment.

Formula	☄ ☽	Candle Color	Candle Type
Purpose			

Equanimity ♃♀ ☾   Green   Taper/Votive
Spell to bring about harmony and good feeling within yourself or another person.

Evoke Love ♃♀ ☾   Pink   Taper/Votive
Spell to bring love into your life.

Exorcism ♄ ☽   Black   Taper/Votive
Spell to purge & banish any & all evil or negative energies in a place or surrounding a person. Use with scent bag & bath crystals.

Expansion ♂ ☾   Red   Taper/Votive
Spell to make your powers & influence larger & more potent.

Faerie Vision ☽ ☺   Silver   Taper/Votive
Spell to see the magickal world of the fairy people. Use with scent bag & bath crystals.

Faith ☽ ☺   White   Taper/Votive
To focus on &/or restore your faith and belief in benevolent higher powers.

Fascination ♆ ☽   Turquoise   Taper/Votive
Spell to fascinate and beguile the object of your affection.

Fast Luck ♀ ☾   Red/Dk. Green/Orange Power 16"
Spell to turn luck from bad to good quickly in a big way.

Fertility ♀ ☾   Green   Taper/Votive
Spell to increase fertility & creativity in body mind or spirit. Use with scent bag & bath crystals.

Fidelity ☽ ☾   Silver/Green   Taper/Votive
             ☺   Male/Female
Do spell work at the waxing moon then put scent bag under your lover's pillow for three days together at the full moon to insure faithfulness.

Focus ♀ ☾   Yellow   Taper/Votive
Spell to improve concentration. Use with scent bag & bath crystals.

Follow Me ♄ ☾   Red Taper/Votive/Male/Female
Spell to entrance & lead the object of your desire.

Foresight ♅ ☺   Blue   Taper/Votive
Spell to increase ability to sense future events and trends.

Formula	☿ ☾	Candle Color	Candle Type
	Purpose		

Forget a Past Love ♄ ☽ Black Taper/Votive/Male/Female
Spell to release an old love & make room for the new.

Forget Me Not ♄ ☿ Gold Taper/Votive
Spell to leave the lasting impression you desire.

Four-Leaf Clover ♀ ☾ Yellow Taper/Votive
Spell to charge a luck charm to be carried on your person or in your purse.

French Love ♀ ☾ Pink Taper/Votive/Male/Female
Spell to evoke swift brief passion for a night or weekend. Use with scent bag & bath crystals to put spice into a love affair.

Friendship ♃♀ ☾ Green Taper/Votive
Spell to draw true and lasting friendship into your life.

Gamblers ♀ ☾ Orange Taper/Votive
Spell to increase the odds in your favor.

Get Rich ♀♃ ☾ Green/Purple Taper/Votive
Spell to bring material wealth and well-being.

Gnomes' Gold ♀ ☾ Orange Taper/Votive
Spell to reveal the hiding place of fairy riches.

Gratitude ☉♃ ☾ Purple Taper/Votive
Spell to insure gratitude for something you have done or given.

Graveyard ♄ ● Black Taper/Votive/Skull
Use in spellwork involving the ancestors & the dead.

Guardian ☽♄ ☾ Purple Taper/Votive/Cat/Snake
Spell to summon a spirit guardian.

Gypsy ♅ ☾ Orange Taper/Votive
Spell to evoke the wild freedom in yourself or someone else. Use with scent bag & bath crystals.

Gypsy Gold ♄ ☾ Yellow Taper/Votive
Spell to help you sort the true from the false.

Happiness ☉ ☾ Yellow Taper/Votive
Spell to promote joy in life. Use with scent bag & bath crystals.

Happy Together ♀ ☾ Green Taper/Votive/Male/Female
Spell to increase & ensure happiness & harmony between two parties.

Formula	♄ ☽	Candle Color	Candle Type	Purpose
Healing	☉ ☽	Red/Blue/Dk Green	Power 16"	Spell to promote healing of mind, body &/or spirit. Use with scent bag & bath crystals.
Helping Hand	♃ ☽	Purple	Taper/Votive	Spell to get help when you need it.
Hex Breaker	♄ ●	Reversible/Red/Black	Power 16"	Spell to banish ill wishing sent by someone else. Use with scent bag & bath crystals.
Higher Consciousness	♃ ○	Purple	Power 16"	Ritual to open yourself to the expanded universe & sense of your place in it. Use with scent bag & bath crystals.
Higher Self	♃ ○	Purple	Taper/Votive	Ritual to open yourself to your highest spiritual self & become consciously aware of its guidance in your life.
Hope	☉ ☽	White	Taper/Votive	Spell to open a heart closed by pain &/or stress to accept new beneficial associations & opportunities. Use with scent bag & bath crystals.
Horn of Plenty	♀ ☽	Green	Taper/Votive	Spell to assure that there is plenty for everyone at a gathering or an occasion.
Hospitality	♀♃ ☽	Green	Taper/Votive	Spell to make your home's atmosphere gracious and pleasing to your guests.
House Blessing	♄ ☽	White/Lavender/Lt. Blue	Power 16"	Spell to insure your living quarters are blessed and protected.
I Am	☉♂ ☽	Red	Taper/Votive	Spell to increase self-confidence & self-esteem. Use with scent bag and bath crystals.
Illusions	♆☿ ☽	Yellow	Taper/Votive	Spell to create or dispel illusions. Use with scent bag & bath crystals
Image Magick	♃♆ ☽	Indigo	Taper/Votive	Spell to enhance power & effectiveness of sympathetic Magick image making, write name of individual the ritual is to represent on the candle.
Immortality	☉ ☽	Gold	Taper/Votive	Spell to insure physical health & vigor & spiritual power. Use with scent bag & bath crystals.

Formula / Purpose	☞ ☽	Candle Color	Candle Type

Improve Relationship ♀♂ ☾   Red Taper/Votive/Male/Female in pair
Write the names of the parties involved on the candle before you anoint it with the oil.

Improve Business ♄ ☾   Green   Taper/Votive
Spell to draw customers and opportunities to expand and improve your business.

Increase Fertility ♀ ☾   Green   Taper/Votive
Spell to increase fertility in body, mind or spirit.

Increase Income ♃ ☾   Green   Taper/Votive
Spell to secure and magnify increased cash flow.

Increase Marital Bliss ♂♀ ☾   Red   Taper/Votive
Spell to reawaken & intensify joy in a marriage or loving partnership. Use with scent bag and bath crystals.

Increase Perception ♀ ☾   Yellow   Taper/Votive/Skull
Spell to awaken senses on all levels. Use with scent bag & bath crystals.

Incubus, Get Rid of ♅ 🌑   Black   Taper/Votive
Spell to banish annoying male spiritual sexual entity. Use with scent bag & bath crystals.

Inspiration/Creativity ♀♀ ☾   Yellow   Taper/Votive
Spell to awaken creative inspiration. Use with scent bag and bath crystals.

Instant Money ♆ ☾   Green   Taper/Votive
Spell to bring about instant inflow of cash.

Irresistible ☉ ☾   Gold   Taper/Votive
Spell to make someone irresistible to the object of one's desires. Use with scent bag and bath crystals.

Job Opportunity ☉ ☾   Orange   Taper
Spell to find a good job use with bath crystals & scent bag

Journey of the Heart ☉ ☾   Orange   Taper/Votive
Spell to encourage love, truth and insight between a couple all with peace.

Just Judge ♃ ☾   Purple   Taper/Votive
Spell to insure a just and fair hearing by an impartial judge.

Justice ♃ ☾   Purple   Taper/Votive
Spell to insure that justice is carried out.

Keep a Lover Home ♀ ☾   Pink Taper/Votive/Male/Female
Binding spell to keep a lover true.

Formula	☄ ☾ Purpose	Candle Color	Candle Type

Knowledge ☿ ☾ — Yellow — Taper/Votive
Spell to gain the knowledge you want and need.

Law Stay Away ♄☿ 🌑 — Indigo — Taper/Votive
Spell to gain immunity from the notice of legal matters.

Leprechaun's Wish ♀ ☾ — Rainbow — Taper/Votive
Spell to gain a favor from the fairy folk.

Let Me Go ☾♄ 🌑 — Black — Taper/Votive
Spell to release someone from any & all ties with and control by a group or individual.

Life After Death ♄ ☾ — White/Black — Taper/Votive/Skull
Spell to increase knowledge & awareness of the Other Side.

Longevity ☉ ☾ — Orange — Taper/Votive
Spell to increase physical health and vigor. Use with scent bag and bath crystals.

Lottery ☿ ☾ — Yellow — Taper/Votive
Spell to increase chances of winning the lottery.

Love ♀ ☾ — Red/Pink/White — Power 16"
Spell to wake passion, desire and genuine caring. Use with scent bag and bath crystals.

Love Be Sweet ♀ ☾ — Pink — Taper/Votive
Spell to evoke gentleness and tenderness in a relationship. Use with scent bag and bath crystals.

Love Everlasting ♀ ☾ — Pink — Taper/Votive
Spell to bring true and lasting love and fidelity into your life. Use with scent bag and bath crystals.

Love is the Law ♀ ☾ — Pink — Taper/Votive
Spell to cause the law of brotherhood and harmony to prevail.

Love Letters ☿ ☾ — Yellow — Taper/Votive
Spell to encourage a loved one to send loving messages in writing.

Love Lies Bleeding ♀☉ ☾ — Pink/Green — Taper/Votive
Ritual to heal a broken heart. Use with bath crystals and scent bag.

Lover Come Back ☾ ☾ — White — Taper/Votive/Male/Female
Write the name of the straying loved one on the candle. Use with scent bag and bath crystals.

Lovers ♀ ☾ — Red — Taper/Votive Male/Female in pairs
Spell to unite two people in a loving relationship.

Formula	⚸ ☽ Purpose	Candle Color	Candle Type

Lust ♂ ☾ Red Taper/Votive
Spell to bring about passion. Use with scent bag and bath crystals.

Luv Luv Luv ♂♀ ☾ Pink Taper/Votive
　　　　　　　　　　Green Male/Female
Spell to draw a passionate and joyful love affair. Use with scent bag and bath crystals.

Magnetic (for Men) ♂♃ ☉ Red Taper/Votive
Spell to increase someone's sexual attractiveness to draw a lover or mate. Use with scent bag and bath crystals.

Magnetic (for Women) ♀♃ ☉ Green Taper/Votive
Spell to increase someone's sexual attractiveness to draw a lover or mate. Use with scent bag and bath crystals.

Making Up ☽ ☾ White Taper/Votive/Male/Female
Spell to bring about a reconciliation.

Manifestation ♄ ☉ Purple Taper/Votive
Spell to cause the object of your desire to come into physical reality.

Massage #1
　　　Select the planetary influence and color taper or votive candle most appropriate to your purpose charge by the moon to draw out and ground negative, unhealthy energies or to charge with desired positive energy. A relaxing fragrance to charge with your healing intention.

Massage #2
　　　A stimulating fragrance to charge with your healing intention.

Meditation ☽ ☉ White Taper/Votive
Ritual to deepen and clarify the level of meditation. Use with scent bag and bath crystals if desired.

Medium's Oil ♄☿ ☾ Indigo/Yellow Taper/Skull
Spell to open the spirit to other plane vibrations and allow them to communicate with this plane. Use with scent bag and bath crystals.

Mend a Broken Heart ♂♀ ☾ Pink/Green Taper
Spell to ease the pain of loss and start the healing process. Use with scent bag and bath crystals.

67

Formula	☿ ☽ Purpose	Candle Color	Candle Type

Mental Power ☿ ☾ Yellow/White Taper/Cat/Snake
Spell to increase focus, clarity and retention use with scent bag and bath crystals.

Money ♃ ☾ Green/Gold/Red Power 16"
Spell to draw in ready cash. Use with scent bag and bath crystals.

Mourning ♄ ☽ Black Taper
Ritual to commemorate one who has passed over and ease the grieving process for those left behind.

Move, Neighbor ♄ ☾☽ Red Taper/Votive
Spell to encourage troublesome neighbors to move somewhere else quietly and quickly.

Musician's Oil ♀ ☾ Pink Taper/Votive
Spell to help the musician's instrument be in tune, the voice in tune with the instrument and the song in tune with the audience. Use with scent bag and bath crystals.

Necromancy ♄ ☽ White Taper/Votive/Skull
Spell to communicate with the dead.

Neutralizing ♄ ☽ Black Taper/Votive
Spell to neutralize and dispel negative influences on any level. Use with scent bag and bath crystals.

New Aeon ♀ ☾ Lavender Taper/Votive
Spell to encourage connection to the energies of the coming New Age.

New Beginnings ♃ ☾ Purple Taper/Votive
Lavender
Mauve
Spell to help find a fresh start in any area of your life. Use with scent bag and bath crystals.

Night Light ☽ ☉ White Taper/Votive
Spell to give comfort in the night, in case of nightmares or fear of the dark. Charge candle at full of moon. Use bath crystals before retiring, place scent bag under pillow.

Old Self ☉ ☾ Gold Taper/Votive
Spell to bring an individual back into focus and familiarity after a time of great stress and change. Use with scent bag and bath crystals.

Optimist ♃☉ ☾ Yellow Taper/Votive
Spell to help see the brighter side of things.

Formula ☞ ☽ Purpose	Candle Color	Candle Type

Oracle ☿ ☾   Yellow   Taper/Votive/Skull
Spell to open the mind to receive psychic predictions.

Out of Body Experience ♀ ☾   Blue   Taper/Votive
Spell to safely assist the spirit in letting go of the body to travel to other planes. Use with scent bag and bath crystals.

Over Sea Safety ☽♆ ☾   White   Taper/Votive
Spell to insure protection and safety for someone who goes over the ocean on travels in foreign countries.

Partings ♄ ☾   Black   Taper/Votive
Spell to ease partings & separations. Use with scent bag and bath crystals.

Passion ♂ ☉   Red   Taper/Votive/Male/Female
Spell to arouse passion in a lover. Use with scent bag & bath crystals.

Past Lives ♆ ☾   Indigo   Taper/Votive
Spell to help recall lifetimes clearly and without emotional entanglement.

Peace ♀ ☾   Green   Taper/Votive
Spell to soothe the mind and spirit.

Peace of Mind ♃ ☾   Purple   Taper/Votive
Spell to soothe the mind and spirit especially with the knowledge that everything that could be done has been done.

Peaceful Sleep ♆ ☾   White/Turquoise   Taper/Votive
Spell to give peaceful and restful sleep. Charge candle at full of moon. Use bath crystals before retiring place scent bag under pillow.

Perseverance ♂ ☾   Red   Taper/Votive
Spell to insure inner strength & courage. Use with scent bag and bath crystals.

Positive Vibrations ☉ ☉   White   Taper/Votive
Spell to draw beneficial energy. Use with scent bag & bath crystals.

Power ☉♂ ☾   Red   Taper/Votive
Spell to access your own inner powers. Use with scent bag and bath crystals.

Formula	☞ ☽ Purpose	Candle Color	Candle Type

Power Hand Wash ☉ ☽ Red Taper/Votive
Spell to use before healing with your hands put a few drops of the oil in a basin of heated water to wash hands.

Promotion ☉ ☾ Orange Taper/Votive
Spell to get a better job use with scent bag and bath crystals.

Prophetic Dreams ☽ ☽ Indigo Taper/Votive/Skull
Write the question you want answered on the candle sleep with the candle lit in your bedroom each night for the three days of the full moon. Use bath crystals before retiring.

Prosperity ♀♃ ☾ Dk Green Power 16"
Moss Green
Yellow
Spell to draw riches and plenty on all levels.

Protect a Child ☽ ☾ Green Taper
Spell to protect a child from physical and spiritual danger. Charge a charm or scent bag if desired. Use with bath crystals.

Protect the Home ☽♄ ☾ Green Taper
Spell to guard the home against all forms of negativity and intrusion.

Protection ☽ ☾ Green/Gold/White Power 16"
General safety spell for persons, objects & places. Use with scent bag and bath crystals.

Protection Against Fascination ☽♄ ☾ Green Taper/Votive
Spell for psychic protection.

Psychic Development ☿ ☾ Purple Taper/Skull
Spell to become in tune with all your inner senses and awareness.

Purify a Sick Room ☉ ☾ Purple Taper
Spell to clear out the negativity brought on by disease or injury.

Rainfall ☽♅ ☾ Blue Taper/Votive
Spell to evoke the feeling of a gentle rainfall. Useful in weather magick.

Reality ♄ ☾ Indigo/White Taper/Votive
Spell to dispel delusion and illusion. Use with scent bag and bath crystals.

Formula ☞ ☽ Purpose	Candle Color	Candle Type

Rebirth ☽ ☾   Purple   Taper/Votive
Spell to bring someone into a new life after putting the old one to rest. Use with scent bag and bath crystals.

Reconciliation ☽♀ ☾   Green   Taper/Votive Male/Female in pair
Spell to bring disagreeing parties together amicably.

Regain Passion ♂ ☉   Red   Taper/Votive Male/Female
Spell to put the spark back in a relationship. Use with scent bag and bath crystals.

Relaxation ♀ ☾   Lt. Blue   Taper/Votive
Spell to leave your cares and stress behind for a while. Use with scent bag and bath crystals.

Remind Him of You ♀ ☾   Yellow Taper/Votive/Male/Female
Spell to cause someone to think of you. Use with scent bag and bath crystals.

Repel Jealousy ♄ ☽   Purple   Taper/Votive
Spell to turn away jealousy from you in love, work or life. Use with scent bag and bath crystals.

Return to Me ☽ ☾   Red   Taper Male/Female
Spell to bring back someone who is gone from you.

Reunite ☽ ☾   White   Taper/Votive Male/Female in pair
Spell to bring two people together again.

Reversing ♄ ☉   Red / Black / White   Power 16"
Powerful spell to turn away all negativity, ill wishing and harm. Use with scent bag & bath crystals.

Safe Journey ☽   White   Taper/Votive
Spell to assure safety and ease of travel. Use with scent bag and charm of your choice.

Seance ♀ ☾   Yellow   Taper/Votive Skull, Cat or Snake
Spell to make the way open for communication with spirits who reside on other planes.

Seduction ♂♀ ☾   Red Taper/Votive/Male/Female
Spell to seduce the object of your desires. Use with scent bag and bath crystals.

Formula	⊘ ☽ Purpose	Candle Color	Candle Type

See Truth ♀ ☾   Yellow   Taper/Votive
Spell to remove the veil of deceit and illusion so the truth can be known. Can be used with scent bag and bath crystals.

Self-Acceptance ☉ ☾   Orange   Taper/Votive
Spell to increase self-esteem and self-worth. Use with scent bag and bath crystals.

Separation ♄ ☽   Black   Taper/Votive
Spell to separate parties without turmoil.

Serenity ♀ ☾   Lt. Green   Taper/Votive
Spell to develop inner peace and tranquility. Use with scent bag and bath crystals.

Seventh Heaven ♆ ☾   Blue   Taper/Votive
Spell to experience tranquility and bliss beyond this world.

Sexual Potency ♂ ☾   Red   Taper/Male/Female
Spell to increase sexual stamina and desire.

Showers of Gold ♃ ☾   Green/Purple   Taper/Votive
Spell to attract money and riches from all quarters.

Sleep Well ☽♆ ☾   White   Taper/Votive
Spell to insure deep restful sleep. Use bath crystals before retiring. Place scent bag under pillow, light candle in safe place during sleep.

Smudge ☉ ☾   White   Taper/Votive
Spell to cleanse, purify and bless anyone or any environment. Can be used as bath crystals and with scent bag.

Special Wishing ♃ ☾   White   Taper
Write your special wish on the candle before you anoint it with the oil. Use with scent bag and bath crystals.

Spell Binder ♂ ☾   Red   Taper/Votive
Spell to confirm and anchor any magickal workings.

Spirit Caller ♀ ☾   Purple   Taper/Votive/Cat/Snake
Spell to summon spirits.

Spirit Guide ♀ ☾   Purple   Taper/Votive/Cat/Snake
Spell to request a personal spirit guide and establish a sensitivity to communications with your guide. Use with scent bag and bath crystals.

Formula	☊ ☽ Purpose	Candle Color	Candle Type

Spiritual Vibrations ♀ ☾   Purple   Taper/Votive
Spell to cause a higher vibration of energy in yourself or your environment. Use with scent bag and bath crystals if desired.

Stop Gossip ♄ ☽   Black   Taper/Votive
Spell to cause malicious rumors to cease.

Strength ♂ ☾   Orange   Taper/Votive/Dragon
Spell to draw strength from within and power from the universe. Use with scent bag and bath crystals.

Strengthen Mental ☿☉ ☾   Yellow or Orange   Taper
Spell to sharpen mental focus, comprehension and retention. Use with scent bag and bath crystals.

Study ☿ ☾   Yellow   Taper
Spell to increase comprehension of a field of study or interest. Use with scent bag and bath crystals.

Success ☉ ☽   Gold/Orange/Red   Power 16"
Spell to bring success in whatever venture you wish. Use with scent bag and bath crystals.

Success in Arts ☉♀ ☾   Green/Gold   Taper
Spell to bring success in artistic pursuits and in the artistic community. Use with scent bag and bath crystals.

Success in Life ☉ ☾   Gold   Taper/Votive
Spell to bring you success in your worldly, emotional and spiritual pursuits. Use with scent bag and bath crystals.

Successful Party ♃♀ ☽   Green/Purple   Taper
Spell to insure a joyful gathering.

Succubus -Get Rid Of ♄ ☽   Black   Taper/Votive
Spell to banish annoying female spiritual sexual entity. Use with scent bag and bath crystals.

Summoning ♂♀ ☾   Yellow   Taper/Votive/Cat/Snake
General spell of drawing.

Sweet Dreams ☽♆ ☾   White   Taper/Votive
Spell to insure pleasant dreaming. Use bath crystals before retiring. Place scent bag under pillow, burn candle in a safe place while sleeping.

Sympatico ♀ ☾   Green   Taper/Votive
Spell to cause mutual good feeling and understanding between parties.

Formula	⚭ ☽ Purpose	Candle Color	Candle Type

Telepathy ♉ ☾ Indigo Taper/Votive/Skull
Spell to develop the ability to perceive the thoughts of others. Use with scent bag and bath crystals.

Theta ♆ ☾ Purple Taper/Votive
Spell to induce a state of deep dreamless sleep, brain wave activity. Use with scent bag and bath crystals.

Thief Be Gone ♄ ☽ Black Taper/Votive
Spell to be rid of a thief.

Thief Return Goods ♂ ☾ Yellow Taper/Votive
Spell to cause stolen goods to be returned to you.

Third Eye ♀ ☾ Purple Taper/Votive/Skull
Spell to develop psychic powers such as telepathy and clairvoyance.

Trance ♆ ☾ Purple Taper/Votive/Skull
Spell to induce a stable trance level. Use with scent bag and bath crystals.

Tranquility ♀♃ ☾ Purple Taper/Votive
Spell to develop inner peace and tranquillity. Use with scent bag and bath crystals.

Transcendence ♀ ☾ Purple Taper/Votive/Owl
Spell to aid you in rising above a situation, condition or plane of awareness.

Transferring ♀ ☾ Yellow Taper/Votive
Spell for taking energy from one place and putting it in another.

Transformation ♀ ☾ Rainbow Taper/Votive or Power 16"
Powerful spell to assist in total change from inside to outside on all levels.

True Love ♀ ☾ Green/Pink Taper/Votive Male/Female
Spell to draw true love and affection. Use with scent bag and bath crystals.

Truth ♀ ☾ Yellow Taper/Votive
Spell to cause the truth to be revealed.

Unconditional Love ♀ ☾ Green Taper/Votive
Spell to bring about truly spiritual unconditional love.

Understanding ♀ ☾ Yellow Taper/Votive/Owl
Spell to know the elements of an issue and come to true understanding.

Formula ⚸ ☽ Purpose	Candle Color	Candle Type
Unity ♀ ☾	Green	Taper/Votive
Spell to bring what you desire into harmony.		
Universal Love ☉♃ ☾	Green	Taper/Votive
Spell to promote the vision of universal love between all creatures.		
Universal Peace ♀ ☾	White	Taper/Votive
To promote the vision of peace throughout the world.		
Victory ☉♂ ☾	Red/Orange	Taper/Votive/Dragon
Spell to enable you to overcome adversaries and obstacles.		
Vision S ☾	Yellow	Taper/Votive/Skull
Spell to increase the depth and scope of your perception.		
Vitality ☉ ☾	Orange	Taper/Votive
Spell to increase physical health and vigor. Use with scent bag and bath crystals.		
Vivid Dreams ☽ ☿	White	Taper/Votive
Spell to enable you to dream clearly and recall your dreams. Charge oil at full of moon. Use bath crystals before retiring, put scent bag under pillow, burn candle in safe place while sleeping.		
Voodoo ♄ ☽	Indigo	Taper/Votive
Spell to enable you to impose your will on some one else using image magick		
Ward Off Misfortune ☽ ☽	White	Taper/Votive
Spell to banish & protect from bad luck and accident. Use with scent bag and bath crystals.		
Wealth ♃ ☾	Purple/Green	Taper/Votive
Spell to acquire vast riches.		
Win a Court Case ♃ ☾	Yellow	Taper/Votive
Write the case name and number along with the desired winner on the candle before you anoint it with the oil.		
Winning Number ☿ ☾	Yellow	Taper
Light the candle in a safe place before sleeping to dream of a winning number.		

Formula	♄ ☽	Candle Color	Candle Type
Purpose			
Wisdom ♃ ☾		Purple	Taper/Votive/Owl
Spell to gain true insight & wisdom			
X-Ray Vision ♅ ☽		Black	Taper/Votive
Spell to enable you to see into closed spaces.			
Youth ☿ ☾		Yellow	Taper/Votive
Spell to capture the essence of youth. Use with scent bag and bath crystals.			

Ritual

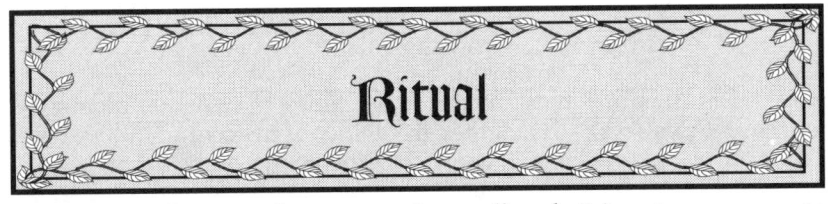

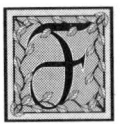

For larger and more complex spellwork, it is not uncommon to work in a ritualized setting. Incense and scented oils play a significant role in any kind of ritual process from the working of a magickal spell to the ceremonial celebration of moons and holidays. While incense fills the air and space around you with magickally charged aromatics, oils can be used for many purposes. The participants can be anointed with oil signifying the purpose of the ritual, the holiday that is being celebrated, or the role they will play in the proceedings. Oil can be used to wash and bless the ritual tools, the altar surface, and even the room in which the ritual takes place. You can even put a couple of drops of special oil on a cotton ball and put it in the drier when you wash the ritual robes so that the fragrance will permeate all through them. Bath crystals can also play a significant part in the ritual process both in preparing the participants to take part in the process of the work or celebration involved by charging and enhancing their personal energy fields to harmonize with the focus or goal of the ritual.

Ritual Formulas

FORMULA	PURPOSE
Altar	To cleanse and consecrate the altar.
Anointing	To anoint and bless the participants. Should be charged at full moon ceremony.
Banishing	To dispel any negative energies or entities.
Bewitched	Enhances spell worked on a person, place or thing.
Black Cat	To invoke the aid of a spirit helper or familiar.
Blessing	To conjure beneficial energy on the recipient.
Ceremony Blessing	Invokes beneficial energy for a ritual ceremony.
Circle	Sets and secure the circle of energy in the ritual.
Commanding	To strengthen the command over energies and entities summoned in the ritual circle.
Cone of Power	To strengthen, focus and enhance the ritually raised vortex of joined power.
Conjuration	To summon and bring about a magickal result; to strengthen and enhance energy as preparation for spell working.
Coven	To bind and focus the energies of a group of individuals who come to contribute their powers to the magickal purpose of the ritual.
Evocation	To raise a specific quality of energy.

Flying	To assist in astral projection and travel.
Grounding	To ground and balance energy in a ritual or the participants.
Handfasting	Bless and bind the joining of two individuals.
High Priest(ess)	To heighten the ability of the central individuals to gather and join the power of the participants for a magickal purpose To balance the energy of one of those individuals should the other not be present.
Holy	To consecrate and bless ritual objects and space.
House Blessing	To seal and bless a house or room after it has been ritually cleansed.
Initiation	To empower the journey of the initiate to gain strength, wisdom and power.
Invocation	To call for a spirit, entity or energy.
Le Sorciere	Formula to enhance and magnify the powers of the spellworker.
Magician's Oil	To draw forth and focus an individual power to do spellwork.
Master	To enhance and magnify the ability of the spell worker to summon and control energies.
Midnight Magick	Tap the energy of the most powerful magick hour.
Pagani	To evoke the spirit of the ancient country people who worshipped the old gods wildly and joyfully in the woods and hills.
Power	Enhances access to the participants strength and energies.
Purification	To remove negativity and inharmonious vibrations. Can be used with bath crystals.
Pre-Ritual	To cleanse and prepare the participants for the ritual. Can be used with bath crystals.
Sacred	To sanctify a person object, space or place. Can be used with bath crystals.
Spell Binder	To confirm and anchor any magickal workings.
Uncrossing	To remove any negative spell work set to bind an individual. Can be used with bath crystals.
Wiccaning	To formalize and celebrate the naming and dedicating of a baby.
Witch's Oil	To strengthen and enhance the individual's power for spellwork and psychic ability.
Witch's Sight	To enhance psychic and magickal perception.
Wizard's Oil	To enhance and strengthen the individual's power to manipulate and manifest energy states.

Celebrations & Sabbats

At special seasons and celebrations of the year a special scent, whether incense or anointing oil, can deepen and enrich the celebration for all participants. Using a specially scented holiday oil can "set the stage" in the ritual area when used before the participants enter. It can also add a gracious ambiance to your home to bring the essence of the season more fully into your daily awareness.

Esbat - A coven meeting that takes place on the night of the full moon

Candlemas - Imbolc - Feb. 2.- The time of blessing and charging the seeds prior to spring planting - lighting candles as a token of the spark of life being held and regenerated

Spring Equinox - Ostara - March 21 - The time of year when the length of the day and night are equal - the festival of rebirth of the earth after the winter's death

Beltane - April 30 - Festival of passion and fertility - lighting of bonfires to dance around to welcome the life fire within - dancing the May Pole

Summer Solstice - June 22 - longest day of the year - The time of power when the sun is strongest, the time for enjoying the first fruits of the season's bounty. A time for asking for abundance, making fertility magick so the harvest will be a fine one.

Lamas - July 31 - The beginning of the Harvest Season honoring grain and the other fruits of the harvest - the mystical symbolism of death and rebirth implied in the harvest

Harvest Moon - The full moon in September - A festival honoring the harvest, a time of Thanksgiving and a reminder to save up all possible resources to last through the winter season.

Autumn Equinox - Sept. 21 - Time of year when the length of the day and night are equal - the Harvest Home or Thanksgiving festival

Hallowmas - Samhain - Oct. 31 - The end of the Harvest Season - the beginning of the pagan winter season at which the dead are honored and put to rest - in some traditions, the New Year's feast

Winter Solstice - Yule - Dec. 22 - longest night of the year - The Yule log reminds us that the fires of life are banked against the coming long sleep of winter, and that even though the worst of the cold days are yet to come, the sun is already returning from his journey south and making each day a little longer. A promise of spring even as winter begins.

Healing & Transformation

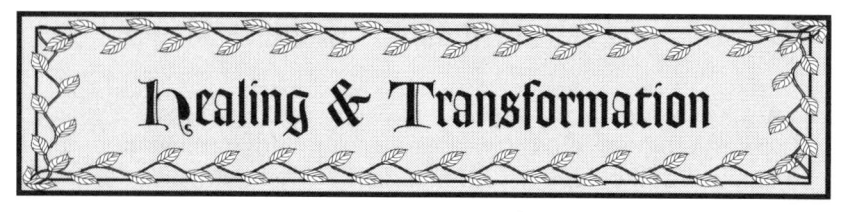

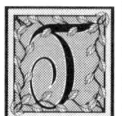

The process you have used for your wish spell can be used for any form of energy work. You can tune your personal energies to a greater harmony and balance with the inner and outer worlds. You can develop your psychic and intuitive talents. You can heal and strengthen yourself and others from the damage left by fatigue, illness and emotional stress and trauma.

The Magick of Color

When spirit manifests itself in the physical universe, it takes the form of energy. Vibration is caused when this energy encounters the resistance inherent in any physical presence. Since no two physical things are exactly the same, no two vibrations are exactly the same. The result is a key signature vibration pattern that is unique to that physical presence. No two vibrations are identical although many are sufficiently similar to appear the same.

You can see this phenomena at work by watching what happens to light encountering a prism. The single ray of light is broken apart changed into a rainbow of color. The spectrum of energy can be seen in many different ways throughout the universe and on our world. Crystals and stones reflect this universal spectrum in their unique key signature vibratory patterns. Each of these patterns also corresponds to color, musical tones on a grander scale and energies within the human body on a more personal scale. The seven visible planets have been used since ancient times to describe this spectrum of energies and how they manifest and interact in our lives. These same energies can be seen in your inner energy system as the Chakra centers.

Your Inner Rainbow

The energies represented by the seven visible planets show themselves in our inner universe as the inner rainbow chain of energy centers called *Chakras*. The Chakra system is much more than a string of etheric Christmas tree lights. These energy centers act as buffers that change the frequency of the energy vibration as the energy passes through the body. There is a constant flow of energy through the system at all times. As the earth energy enters the body through the base or pubic Chakra, each succeeding Chakra it encounters accelerates the vibration of this energy until it passes out of the body at the crown Chakra at the same vibratory rate as the energy entering there. The high vibrational celestial energy goes through the same process as it enters the body at the crown and is successively slower as it passes downward through the Chakras until it exits the system to merge with the earth power.

When a Chakra is blocked or damaged due to injury or trauma, it needs to be cleared and healed in order for the body's energy system to work properly and the organism to be healthy. A process using oils, incense, herbs and candles can attune to the ideal vibration of the Chakra, strengthening the center by supplying the intensified energy to the afflicted area and gently helping to clear the blocked energy.

When the physical body is damaged or impaired due to illness or injury, its energy fields are affected on more than just the physical level. In the same way emotional damage can communicate to the other levels of awareness leaving the individual mentally muddled and physically weakened and more prone to illness. Each level of awareness is connected to the other three, and logically, if there is damage on one level, there is corresponding damage on the others as well. It is only by reaching all the levels of an individual's existence that health and vitality can be restored. This is especially the case if the illness or injury is severe or lengthy. By using incense, oils and bath crystals, the body's energy fields can be encouraged to restore themselves by returning to harmony and balance. The body itself can be helped to, relax and restore its vital resources. Even the surrounding environment can be cleansed of the lingering miasma of sickness and pain and reenergized with healing and soothing vibrations to assist the individual to full recovery. On a deeper level, the energy centers called Chakras can be balanced and restored.

Even if no trauma or injury is involved, it can be a deeply rewarding experience to work with each of your Chakra centers to gain experience of its particular energy and place within the whole of your inner energies. If you feel that one area of your life is not as strong or balanced as you would like it to be you can use Chakra mediation to strengthen and enhance that area and bring it into harmony and balance with the others.

Chakras

Root - Muladhara - Red - The point where the earth energy enters the body. Some say this is located in the center of the pubic bone, others at the base of the spine. The seat of passion and survival instinct. This corresponding stone is garnet or ruby. The energy of this center corresponds to the planet Mars. The powers of this center are sexual enthusiasm and magickal ecstasy. The meditative vision of this Chakra is the lotus with four petals.

Navel - Svadistthana - Orange - The warrior center where identity is realized. This is the center that dictates survival as a personality. It sets boundaries and gives the strength to defend them. This is the womb center where the individual is first nurtured. The corresponding stone is citrine or carnelian. The powers of this center are spiritual strength and magickal courage corresponding to the powers of the sun. The meditative vision is the lotus with 6 petals.

Solar Plexus - Manipura - Yellow - The dancer center, the point of balance and adaptability to change. It rules both instinct and expression. The powers of this center are will power and magnetic force corresponding to the planet Mercury. The corresponding stone is topaz. The meditative vision is the lotus with 10 petals.

Heart - Anahata - Green and Rose - This is the point where the energies meet and are equalized, therefore it is the point at which the angel sits down with the animal in every human being. The point where passion and unconditional love meet. It is the pivot of energies where healing power is generated and expressed. The corresponding stones are Rose quartz and emerald. The power of this center is universal and mystical beauty corresponding to the planet Venus. The meditative vision of this Chakra is the lotus with 12 petals.

Throat - Vishuddhi - Blue - This is the point of force of will, the power of speech. It expresses the strength of the intellect and reason realized in the brow Chakra. The powers of this center are psychic powers and the power of will and expression corresponding to the powers of Saturn. The meditative vision of this Chakra is a lotus with 16 petals. Its corresponding stone is sapphire.

Brow or Third Eye - Ajna - Violet - This is the seat of higher reasoning and ethics. It is the power of spirit encountering the orderly process of reasoning. The corresponding stone is amethyst. The powers of this center are mystical insight and connection to higher awareness corresponding to the planet Jupiter. The meditative vision of the Chakra is the lotus with 2 petals.

Crown - Sahasara - White - This is the point where pure universal spirit energy first encounters the human form. It is the seat of our union with the infinite and it is seen depicted in religious art the world over as a clear flame or halo around an individual's head. The corresponding stone is diamond or moonstone. The power of this center is the transcendental joy of spiritual enlightenment. The meditative vision is a lotus with 1,001 petals. .

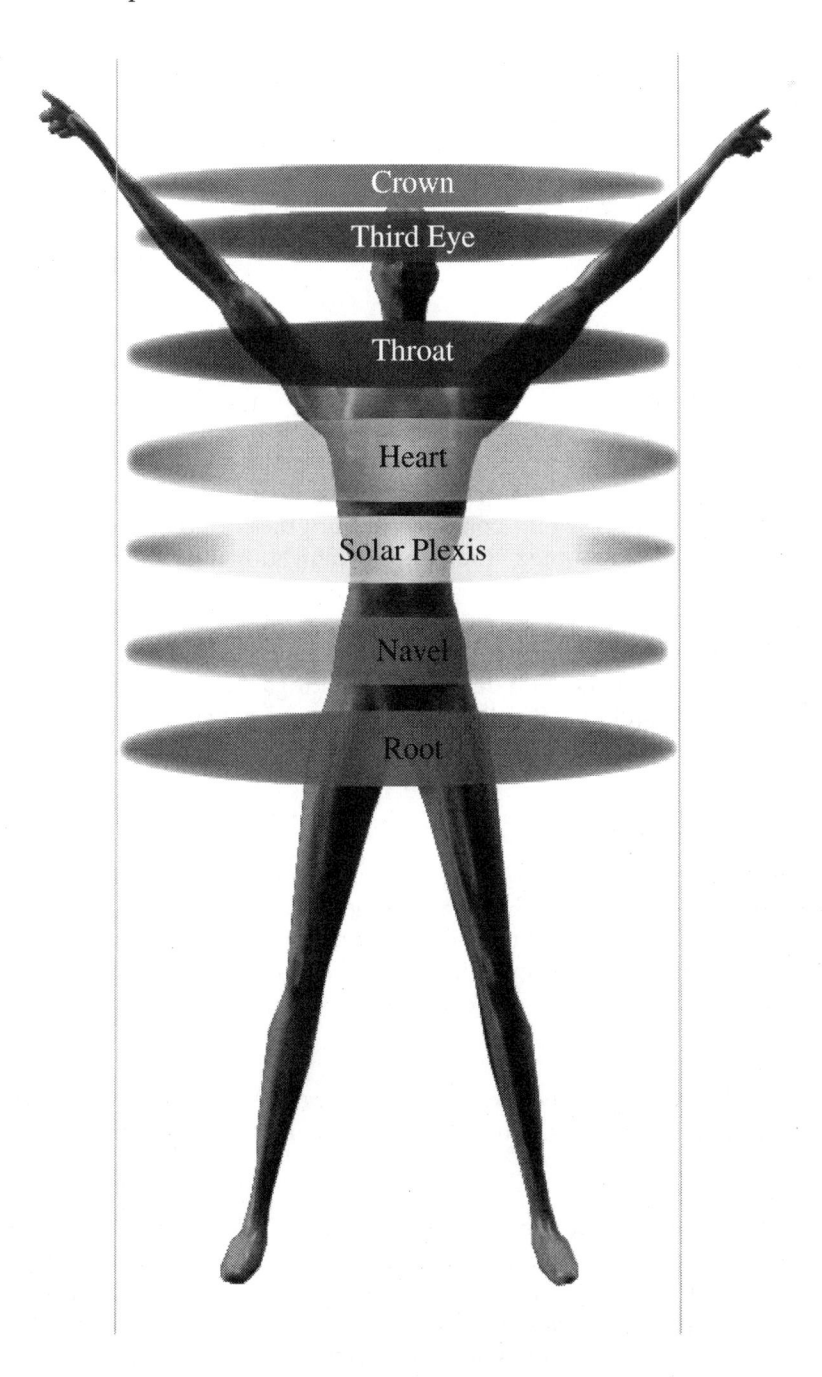

Chakra Healing & Strengthening Process

For this spellworking you will need:

    Candle holder
    Incense burner
    Charcoal block (if you are using powdered incense)
    Candle of the appropriate color
    Oil blended for the Chakra you are working with
    Incense of the same fragrance as the anointing oil

- 1 -

Anoint a candle of the appropriate color with the specified oil in the manner described above, then place it in a holder and light it.

- 2 -

From the flame of this candle, light an incense charcoal block and place it in a dish or sea shell with sand in the bottom (so the heat of the charcoal does not crack the container or burn the surface underneath). Then sprinkle some of the incense on the glowing charcoal.

- 3 -

Move the incense burner so that you are surrounded with a cloud of scented smoke. Draw it deep into your lungs. Let the incense surround you and fill you. Breathe in its energy and essence. Then, anoint the desired Chakra with the same oil with which you dressed the candle.

- 4 -

Now allow the sensation of the glowing candle and the stimulating and relaxing fragrance of the oil and incense to draw you into a relaxed and meditative state. Let your mind quietly fill with the image of the Chakra's lotus vision. Remain in a quiet meditative state for as long as is comfortable.

- 5 -

When you are done, extinguish the candle with your dampened fingers or with a snuffer. Repeat this process as needed.

- 6 -

As you work with these energies, it may be helpful to wear a piece of cloth or cotton ball that has the Chakra oil on it somewhere on your person. You may put it in your pocket or tie it into a scent bag around your neck so that the essence of your work will linger and continue to stimulate your process on a subtle level throughout the day.

The Universe of Spirit & Archetypes

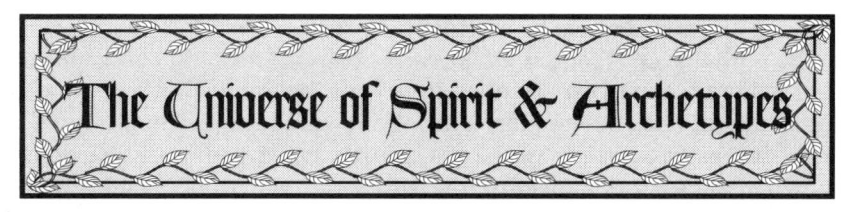

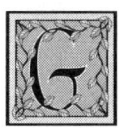

Gods, goddesses, myths, legends, ideals - these are all powerful image energy forms that have reflected the many levels of the human awareness since the beginning of time. The tales human beings have told about the forces of creation and heroic endeavor have come from the deep well springs of the inner consciousness and reflect much about the inner spirit of humankind. They tell of our worst fears, our finest ideals and our greatest aspirations. The faces humankind has painted in myth and religion for its deities tells much about human beings as they have perceived themselves and as they wish to be. These are more than just stories and allegories made up to explain events or invented to entertain the populace. They are reflections of deep human awareness of spiritual realities that defy description or definition by any other means. By examining the myths and stories about humanity's gods and heroes, you can reach beyond the intellect and involve the deeper levels of your consciousness in experiencing and understanding the issues involved. The god and goddess forms in the ancient tales are representative, not only of consciously aware higher beings, but also of archetypal energy states. The portrayals of heroes, heroines and villains say much about that most illusive and ever changing archetype - human beings themselves. The ancient myths describe their constant interaction and the effect these interactions have on the lives of everyday people and the world in which they live.

These legendary and mythical energies exist in what are called Thought Forms. Thought forms are composites of energy of a particular vibration. Over a great length of time so many different people believed in them, prayed and sacrificed to them and told the stories of these gods and heroes that the energy of their belief and passion took on a life and existence all its own. These energies continue to exist today as part of the universal consciousness in which we all participate. You are always connected to the greater universal consciousness. Because you are part of the spiriutal consciousness of humankind, you are also part of and connected to these energies that have been part of the human consciousness since the earliest times. These connections are sleeping inside you and can be awakened and enhanced through spellwork and meditation. The wisdom of kings, the courage of heroes, the cleverness of heroines, the essence of archetypal god forms and many more are part of our inner awareness. By working in the same way you did for wish spells and chakra work, you can connect with these complex energies. You can summon their essences and invite these entities to work on your behalf.

You can experience them, learn from them and awaken this energy as it exists within you. Fragrances, incenses, bath oils, colors and candles will help you tune your own subtle energy fields to align with these greater thought form energies. The following is a simple ritual suggestion. If you wish you may also include a scented bath to infuse your aura and skin with the energy fragrance. You may do this before you proceed with the candle spell or after you complete your meditation but before the candle burns itself out. As with your wish spell, the use of bath crystals will greatly enhance the strength and clarity of the energy you are working with. You may also include incense as you take your energy bath if you chose. This will put you in touch with the energies as they exist within you and in the find their resonance in the greater universe.

Spiritual Magick

For this spellworking you will need:
Candle holder
Incense burner
Picture, artifact, crystal or stone
1 central candle to represent the energy, entity or deity you wish to draw or develop
1 charcoal block (if you are using powdered incense)
1 bottle anointing oil corresponding to the energy, entity or deity
1 package of bath crystals in the same scent as the oil and incense (if desired)

- 1 -

Select the energy you wish to work with. It can be a god, goddess, mythical character or historical figure. Find out as much as you can about this individual then select a picture or object that feels most like this energy. As before, it can be a picture, artifact, crystal or stone.

- 2 -

Dress a candle of the appropriate color with the oil corresponding to the energy you wish to draw. Mark the candle with the name of the entity. While you are doing so, concentrate on the quality of energy you wish to draw and develop within yourself.

- 3 -

Place the candle in the holder and light it. Place the artifact, picture or stone in front of the candle so that the light is reflected on it. Light the incense or charcoal block from the candle and place it in the holder.

- 4 -

Move the incense burner so that you are surrounded with a cloud of scented smoke. Draw it deep into your lungs. Let the incense surround you and fill you. Breathe in its energy and its essence. Then, anoint your forehead and your heart with the same oil that you used to anoint the candle.

- 5 -

Focus your awareness on the artifact representing the energy. Allow the flickering light of the candle to stimulate your inner awareness. Feel the energy of the entity you seek hover before you. Be aware of its nearness. Now you can feel an answer stirring inside you. You begin to feel a corresponding energy resonate within you. Let the experience fill you. Let your mind quietly fill with the awareness of the power of this energy. Continue in this meditative state until you feel comfortable with your connection to this energy.

- 6 -

When you are done, extinguish the candle with your dampened fingers or a snuffer. Repeat the ritual as often as you feel the need.

- 7 -

As you work with these energies, it may be helpful to wear a piece of cloth or cotton ball anointed with the scented oil somewhere on your person. You may put it in your pocket or tie it into a scent bag around your neck so that the energy and essence of your work will linger and continue to stimulate your inner awareness throughout the day. You might also find it helpful to carry a token, image or crystal that you consciously connect with this energy to contribute to the connection process.

Spiritual Formulas
African Powers

The powerful and benevolent spirits of the Yoruban religion, called Orishas, whose worship was brought to the New World with the slave trade, now celebrated and revered through much of North and South America.

Ellugua / Eshu - Youngest of the Orishas, trickster through whom all messages and offerings must pass. Power of the crossroads. His colors are black and red.

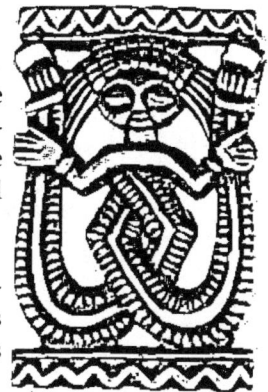

Babalu-Aye - Crippled healer orisha symbolized by the crutches he walks with, possessor of all medical and healing lore. His colors are violet and white.

Chango - Great worldly king, greatest of lovers, feasters, fighters, and drinkers. He is the magnificent drummer and dancer. His colors are red and white.

Obatala - The Pure White King creator of earth from the waters, father of all the other Orishas, cool personification of order, reason and peace. His color is white.

Ochosi - Hunter; lord of justice and law; tireless tracker who never loses sight of his quarry. His colors are blue and yellow.

Ogun - Master of crafts especially metal smithing, inventions and progress. He rules all things of iron and steel tools, weapons and also the surgeon's blade. His colors are green and black.

Oshun - Goddess of Rivers and All Fresh Waters, Joyful mistress of love, beauty, pleasure and dancing, the African Aphrodite. Her colors are gold and white.

Oya / Yansa - Wild woman of the whirlwind, beautiful warrior goddess, bringer of changes, patroness of the market place. Her colors are plum purple and the rainbow.

Yemaya - The Ocean Mother; beautiful and loving mother of all creatures who holds limitless wealth in her depths; mother of infinite compassion. Her colors are blue and white.

Angels

Angels are the messengers or mediators between humankind and the divine archetypal energies of creation. Angels can give help in daily life or provide special energy and assistance in magickal workings. According to ancient Judeo-Christian belief, all things existing in Creation have a presiding angel or personification of its divine life force.

Angels of Air - Chasan, Casmaron, Cherub, Iahmel

Angels of Earth - Azriel, Admael, Arkiel, Arciciah, Ariel, Harabael, Yabbashael

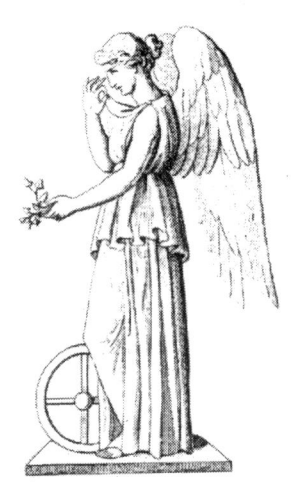

Angels of Fire - Nathaniel, Arel, Atuniel, Jehoel, Ardarel, Gabriel, Seraph

Angels of Water - Tharsus, Arariel, Talliud, Phul, Michael, Anafiel

Cherubim - Bearer's of God's throne; personifications of the winds who unceasingly praise their Maker

Guardian Angel - It is said that every person has a Guardian Angel who watches over them. This fragrance is used in seeking to make closer contact with that angel or when asking that angel for advice and assistance on a particular issue such as a healing or a life crisis.

Michael - The greatest of all the Angels; also, patron of Policemen

Seraphim - The highest order of angels; the angels of love, light and fire

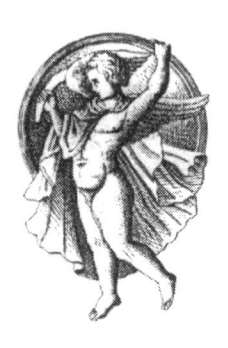

Enochian

Each unit of time was attended by its own angel because units of time were considered manifestations of Divine Order. It is common in ceremonial magickal practice to appeal to the angels who represent the appropriate day and hour when the magickal work is taking place. The oils can be used to anoint altar candles if specific ones are being used for these spirits or the appropriate incense pertaining to each entity can be lighted or dropped onto the charcoal as each angel is named and summoned.

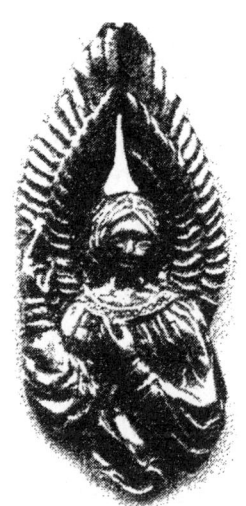

MONTHS

Gabriel (January)
Barchiel (February)
Machadiel (March)
Asmodel (April)
Ambrirel (May)
Muriel (June)
Verchiel (July)
Hamaliel (August)
Uriel (September)
Barbiel (October)
Adnachiel (November)
Hanel (December)

SEASONS

Spugliguel (Spring)
Tubiel (Summer)
Torquaret (Autumn)
Attarib (Winter)

WEEKDAYS

Gabriel (Monday)
Kahmael (Tuesday)
Raphael (Wednesday)
Tzaphkiel (Thursday)
Haniel (Friday)
Cassiel (Saturday)
Raphael (Sunday)

FOUR DIRECTIONS

Gabriel (East)
Raphael (West)
Michael (South)
Uriel (North)

Tree of Life (Kaballah)

The Kabalistic Tree of Life represents a schematic of the paths that spiritual energy takes as it proceeds from its entry into this Universe, becoming more solid until it finally manifests on this physical plane of reality. Each stage it passes through is called a "sephiroth" which translates from the Hebrew as "divine emanation". Each Sephiroth is identified with a planet and is in turn personified by an angelic presence that embodies the essence of the abstract condition that the sephiroth represents.

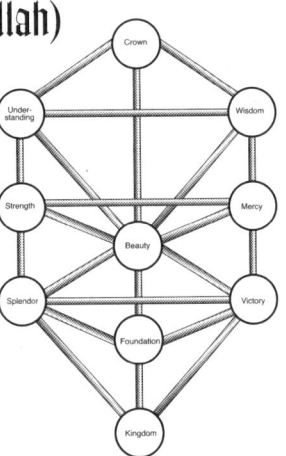

Binah - Understanding - Saturn ♄ - Tzaphkiel

Chesed - Mercy, Greatness - Jupiter ♃ - Tzadkiel

Chokmah - The Zodiac - Uranus ♅ - Ratziel

Da'ath - Knowledge, Invisible - Sephirah

Geburah - Strength, Justice, Mars ♂ - Khamael

Hod - Glory - Mercury ☿ - Raphael

Kether - Crown, Primum Mobile, Neptune ♆ - Shekinah or Metatron

Malkuth - Kingship - Elements, Earth - Sandalphon

Middle Pillar - The central pillar of the Tree of Life which unites all three and is the direct path of divine energy manifesting into Earthly consciousness - also refers to the current of primal power running through the human body

Netzach - Victory - Venus ♂ - Haniel

Solomon's Wisdom - It is said that Solomon was the greatest of Magicians and through his learning and wisdom brought all angels and demons under his command.

Tiphareth - Beauty - Sol ☉ - Michael

Yesod - Foundation - Luna ☽ - Gabriel

Arthurian

Arthur - Once & future king of Britain (450 AD).

Avalon - The "Isle of Apples" Timeless island of Immortal heroes where Arthur's sword was forged and where he was taken to be healed after the battle at Camlan.

Bediver, Sir - Prominent knight known for his valor and friendship with Arthur who was given the task of casting Arthur's sword Excalibur back into the lake after the last battle.

Camelot - Arthur's court palace; point of departure for Grail Quests; home of the Round Table.

Caradwyg - Hero knight, son of Arthur's niece, Ysave. He won many miraculous contests because of his nobility and purity of heart.

Cauldron of Annun - Magick cauldron from which only the brave & true can eat.

Constantine - Arthur's cousin took up Arthur's crown when both Arthur and Mordred died.

Erec, Sir - Knight who betrayed his vows and blamed his betrayal on his wife, Enid. He put her through many cruel trials to prove her innocence.

Excalibur - Arthur's sword, forged in Avalon and given him by the mystical Lady of the Lake; Some say this was also the sword he drew from the Stone which proved he was the rightful king of Britain.

Fisher King - Wounded King identified with Bran the Blessed, who was the Keeper of the Grail.

Galahad, Sir - Illegitimate son of Lancelot and Elaine who grew up to be the perfect pure and chaste Grail Knight, the epitome of chivalry and spiritual purity.

Gareth, Sir - Son of King of Orkney known as "the Generous" unintentionally slain by Lancelot.

Gawain, Sir - Son of King of Orkney, known for his bravery in combat, killed in battle with Mordred, Arthur's knight.

Glastonbury - Part of Avalon, Arthur's resting place; Ancient pagan holy site with Labyrinthine walk of initiation; most ancient site of Christianity in Britain, founded by Joseph of Arimathea when he brought the Grail to Britain.

Guinevere - Arthur's wife and queen, lover of Lancelot, whose infidelity began the dissolution and downfall of the Round Table.

Gwendydd - Merlin's Sister.

Holy Grail - Cup used at Last Supper by Jesus; object of the Grail Quest; mystical symbol of the Cauldron of Death and Rebirth.

Isle of Annun - Land of the Dead.

Kay, Sir - Arthur's seneschal and foster brother, killed in France in battle.

Lady of Shallot - Elaine, mistress of Lancelot, mother of Galahad. Also, Tennyson's poem about Elaine's hopeless love for Lancelot and how she died of a broken heart after giving birth to Lancelot's son.

Lady of the Lake - Variously known as Vivianne, Eviane, Niniene. The keeper of Arthur's sword, who claimed it back again after the last battle. The lover and betrayer of Merlin.

Lancelot - Arthur's favorite knight who rescued Guinevere from her abductors and became her champion and lover; symbol of the greatest and finest worldly knight.

Laudine - Gawain's friend.

Merlin - Arthur's magician, counsellor, seer and tutor, great prophet and mage.

Mordred - Arthur's bastard son by his half sister Morgause. He betrayed Arthur first by setting the knights against one another and engineering the fall of the Round Table, then by openly challenging Arthur for the throne. Arthur killed him but received his own mortal wound from him.

Morgan Le Fey - Faerie queen, sorceress, healer and shape-changer. Eldest and most beautiful of nine sisters living on the Isle of Avalon.

Mt. Badon - Site where Arthur won decisive victory over the Saxons.

Niniene - Merlin's student, lover and betrayer, who enchanted him with spells he taught her, then sealed him in a tomb and stole his power (variant of Eviane, Vivianne, and the Lady of the Lake).

Perceval, Sir - Knight, finder of the Grail, who began as an ignorant clod and gradually learned chivalry and knighthood due to his inherent goodness and naturally honorable nature.

Prydwyn - Arthur's ship.

Round Table, Knights of the - 1,600 men sworn to the principles of defending the weak and helpless, and securing Britain against foreign invasion. They later went on the Quest for the Holy Grail.

Silchester - Arthur's crowning place.

Tintagel - Arthur's birthplace, castle in Cornwall.

Uther Pendragon - Arthur's father who with the help of Merlin took the form of the King of Cornwall in order to sleep with Igraine his wife. After the death of the king of Cornwall that night, Uther married Igraine who bore him Arthur.

Vivianne - Merlin's student, lover and betrayer, who enchanted him with spells he taught her then sealed him in a tomb and stole his power (variant of Eviane, Vivianne, and the Lady of the Lake).

Yvain, Sir - Last of the knights to die in the final battle before the death of the King himself.

Assyro-Babylonian Deities

Anshar - Sumerian god of the Celestial World; the first primal male principle of Creation.
Anat (Qadesh) - Warlike goddess of Desire called Mother of Nations, consort of Baal, rode to battle on a lion.
Antum - Goddess, wife and female counterpart of the sky god, Anu.
Anu - Mesopotamian God of Heaven.
Apsu - Babylonian abyss, The primordial waters which surround and support Creation.
Astarté - Lady of Byblos, oldest Great Mother Goddess of the Middle East; also identified with the planet Venus.
Bel/Baal - General term meaning "Lord" or "Lord of", generally a sky or fertility god.
Damkina - Babylonian Lady of the Earth, wife of Ea, God of the Sweet Waters.
Dagon - God of ancient Ashdod, half-man/half-fish.
Habur - Variant of Eridu, second capitol of Sumeria before the Deluge.
Haddad - God of the Atmosphere, Clouds and Storms; Rain-giver, Thunder-bringer; symbol is the bull.
Inanna - Queen of Heaven, Lady of the Horned Moon who grieved over her lost love, Tammuz, so much she went to fetch him from the Underworld.
Ishtar - Babylonian goddess of Venus, the morning star, goddess of love and beauty; also goddess of war who rode a lion into battle.
Kadi - Babylonian Goddess of Justice symbolized the living earth itself on which all oaths were sworn, shown as a snake with a human head.
Kingu - Mesopotamian god whose blood Marduk took to mix with clay and fashion the first human beings.
Marduk - Great God of Babylon; the fertilizing force of water, Creator of the Physical World; Controller of the Destinies of Human Beings.
Namtar - Negative aspect of Fate; bringer of disease to Earth.
Nuah - Meaning "He of Long Life", variant of Noah.
Nusku/Gibil - Assyrian Fire God; sat in judgment over the souls of men who in life had been unjust judges.
Ramman - Assyrian weather god - Thunderer - Pomegranate sacred to him
Tammuz/Dumuzi - Harvest/vegetation god of Mesopotamia; consort of Inanna, King of the Underworld.
Tiamat - Goddess of the Primal Abyss who took the form of a dragon; mother of all the gods of Mesopotamia.

British and Celtic Deities

Adraste - Goddess of War
Aefen/Aife - Princess of the land of Shadows consort of Manawydan, she stole the secret of the alphabet to give to humankind and was changed into a crane as punishment
Brigantia - Celtic "the High One"; sometimes equated with Brigit
Brigit - Virgin goddess of poets, smithcraft and healing, keeper of the Sacred Fire
Britannia - Patron goddess archetype of the Isle of Brittany
Campestres, The / Matres, The / Idises, The - Three Mothers holding bread, fruits and/or a child personifying the ancestor mothers of a family; triple goddess of fertility and abundance
Cernunnos - Horned God of Virility, Lord of the Animals, Stag Lord
Dahut - Pagan priestess and mistress of the drowned city of Ys
Eostre - Goddess of Spring, symbolized by a Hare
Epona - Celtic Goddess of Horses, Abundance & Fertility
Essus - Gallic god of unknown association; said to drink human blood; associated with a bull and three cranes
Godiva - Form of the Goddess who on May Eve rode naked through the countryside to renew her virginity.
Gog - Name for any colossal figure of pagan deity
Grannos - Gallic god of healing connected with hot springs
Herne - British variant of Cernunnos, Lord of the Animals and Forests
Latis - Mother of the World Egg and the Sun
Leucetios/Mars Leucetios - god of war
Llud - Variant of Nuada; leader of the Tuatha da Dannan; Wealth-bringer; Cloud-maker; bringer of Fertility and Healer of the Maimed
Morgan - Variant of Morigan
Morigan - Triple Goddess, Queen of Ghosts; Goddess of War, Crone aspect of the triple goddess
Nemontana - Celtic goddess often coupled with Camulos, god of war, healing & fertility; her name means "she who is revered in the shrine" or "spirit of the sacred grove"
Nixes - Prophetic spirits of the waters, river mermaids
Segomo - Gallic War God
Setlocenia - Goddess of Long Life
Tarvos Trigaranos - Gallic god of unknown association shown with a bull with three cranes on its back like that of Essus
Titania - Name for Diana in her role as Queen of the Faerie Realm
Verbeia - Goddess of the River Wharfe

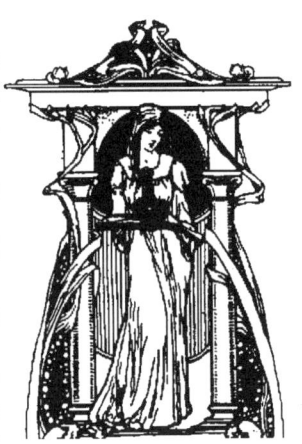

Christian

St. Anthony (of Padua) - Invoked to help find lost objects, Feast Day June 13.

St. Jude Thaddeus - Patron of difficult or lost causes, Feast Day Oct. 28.

St. Michael - Defender of the World Order, Patron of Policemen.

St. Rita - The saint of desperate cases, Feast Day May 22.

Holy Mother - Blessed Virgin, Mother of Jesus, Queen of Heaven.

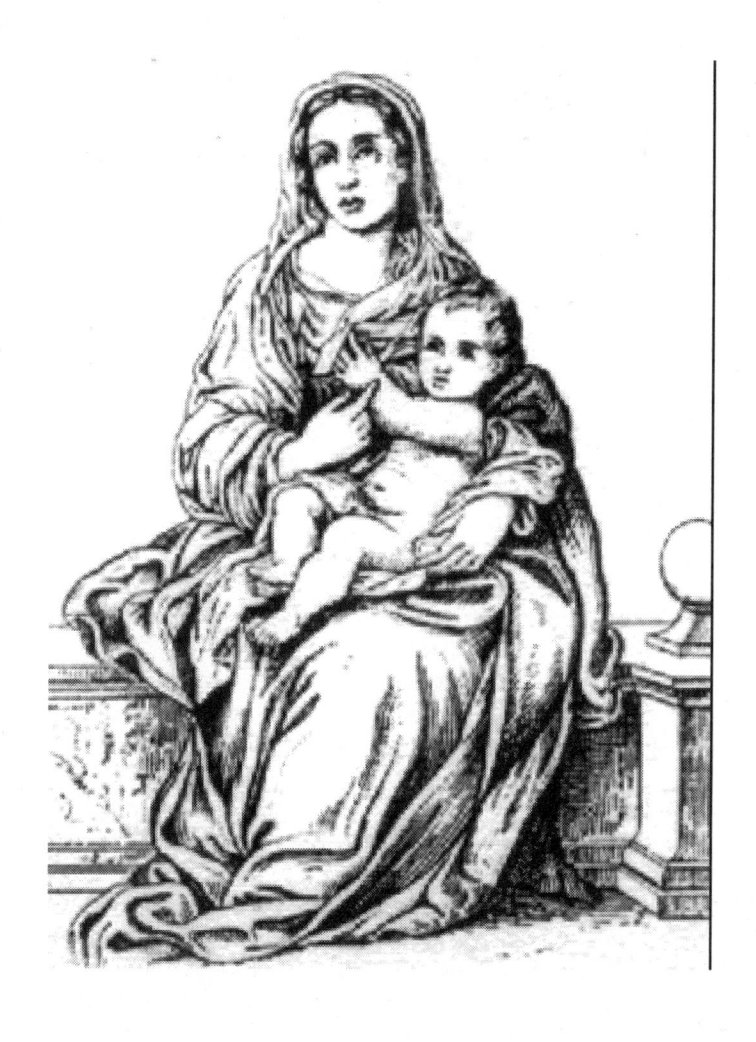

Egyptian Deities And Essences

Aker - Guardian lion of the horizon. The twin guardians (Akeru) guardian of the gates of evening and morning through which the sun-boat passed on its daily journey.

Amemet - Goddess of the Land of the West.

Amon - Called "the Hidden One", supreme unknowable power and creator of the universe.

Amon Ra - The god Amon personified in the Sun.

Anubis - God of Embalming and tombs, guide of the dead through the Underworld, son of Osiris and Nephthys.

Anuket - Called the Embracer, goddess of the rocky river banks and Nile cataracts, wife of the god Knum.

Apep/Apophis - Demon enemy of the Sun, personification of darkness, storm and night who sought to destroy creation.

Atum-Re - Evening aspect of the Sun god Re, the sun on the western horizon, progenitor of the human race.

Ba-Neb-Djedet - Ram god who opened the way for arbitration and mediation between Horus and Set, personification of reason and levelheadedness.

Bast - Cat goddess personifying the fertilizing and nurturing force of the sun. Rules pleasure, dancing, music and joy.

Benu - The Phoenix, pictured as a heron, one of the souls of Ra; mythical fire bird who burst into flames that consumed it, then recreated itself and rose from its own ashes every thousand years.

Bes - Happy fat dancing dwarf god. Patron of women, especially those in childbirth and by association children, cosmetics. Protector from snakes and scorpions.

Cleopatra - Last independent queen of Egypt who captivated both Julius Caesar and Mark Anthony with her beauty and intelligence.

Dedwen - God of Incense - sometimes shown as a lion.

Djet - Symbol of Osiris as the stabilizing strength of the earth and the physical universe. Used as a talisman for strength and health.

Duat - The Underworld below the Earth where the sun god, in his boat, traveled each night.

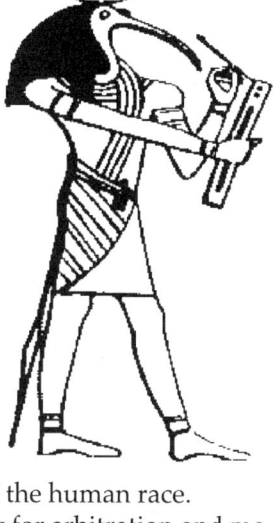

Duamutef - One of the four sons of Horus. Jackal headed Canopic guardian of the stomach. Corresponding to the function of Transmutation. God of the Northern pillar of the physical world and the element Earth.

Geb - God of the physical earth. Who, as a goose, laid the World Egg thereby creating the physical universe.

Hapi - One of the four sons of Horus. Baboon headed Canopic guardian of the Lungs. Corresponding to circulation. God of the Eastern pillar of the physical world and the element Air.

Hathor - Queen of Heaven, Goddess of Love, Mother of Creation, Protector of Women, Mistress of Everything Beautiful.

Heket - Frog goddess of creation & childbirth.

Hetep-Sekhus - Goddess who is identified with the Eye of Ra or with the flame who follows Osiris, who burns up his enemies.

Horus the Elder - Sky God, "Rules with Two Eyes" i.e. the Sun and the Moon brother of Isis, Osiris, Nephthys & Set.

Horus the Younger - Son of Osiris and Isis, Falcon god, defender of home and family who defeated Set, god of Chaos and Storms.

Hu - The personification of the "authoritative utterance" of Ra when giving judgment on the souls of the dead, counterpart of Sia.

Imhotep - Once an historical figure, physician, mathematician, scientist and thought to be the architect of the Step Pyramid, later deified as god of physicians, architects and all learning.

Imset - One of the four sons of Horus Human headed God of the West. Canopic Guardian of the Liver. Corresponding to the function of sorting and the element of water.

Isis - Great Mother Goddess, ideal embodiment of womanhood and motherhood, wife of Osiris, mother of Horus.

Iusas - City in the north, birthplace of the Scarab of the Sun, Khephera.

Kefa - One of the guardians of the corridor of the Tenth Hour of the Night.

Kenemet - Oasis in the Libyan desert, a center for the worship of Amon-Ra.

Khnum - God of Fecundity and Creation, who shapes the body of the fetus in the womb like a potter shapes clay.

Khons - Moon god and god of healing, son of Amon and Mut.

Maahes - Lion headed warrior son of Bast and Ra, personified the scorching heat of the midsummer sun.

Maat/Mayet - Personification of World Order, Truth and Justice, Balance and Harmony on all levels.

Mauet - Ancient variant of the goddess Mut, self-produced; one of the goddesses in the Pyramid Texts.

Mehan/Mahen - Serpent protector who stands upright at the prow of the sun-boat.

Mehuret - A form of mother goddess in whose hall the dead were judged.

Menqet - One of the gods of the Book of the Dead.

Mertseger - She Who Loves Silence. Goddess of the highest mountain in the Valley of the Kings.

Meskhenet - Goddess of Childbirth who appeared at the moment of birth to predict the future of the child.

Mehurt - Goddess Neith as the sacred cow of Creation, Mystical animal mother of the world.

Min - God of Sex, Fecundity and Crops. Also god of roads and travelers.

Montu - Falcon headed God of War.

Mut - Great mother goddess shown variously as a vulture, a cow and a lioness. Wife of Amon.

Nebhet-Hotep - Local variant of Nekhebet, vulture goddess protector of the dead.

Nefertum - Son of Ptah and Sekhmet, Lotus God, personification of the eternal rebirth of creation.

Neith - Ancient goddess of war, archery & weaving.

Nekhbet - Upper Egyptian vulture goddess who along with Uajet the cobra goddess of Lower Egypt, protected the Pharaoh.

Nekhebkau - Snake spirit, protector of Ra's Sun-boat, Lord of Everlasting Time, the Hope of the Dead.

Nefer - Word meaning beautiful, upright and harmonious.

Nephthys - Wife of Set, sister of Isis, Goddess of dreams, divination and all hidden knowledge.

Nu/Nun - Primordial waters of chaos from which the gods arose.

Nut - Sky goddess whose body was the Milky Way. Wife of Geb, Mother of Isis, Osiris, Nephthys and Set.

Osiris - Father of Civilization, Agriculture, and Animal Husbandry, husband of Isis, who was murdered by his brother Seth, then magickally restored to life by Isis, Nephthys and Anubis, He was then transmuted in the Lord of the Underworld, a symbol of the soul's death, destruction and rebirth.

Pakhit - Cat/Lioness goddess whose name means "the Tearer" identified with a vengeful form of Isis.

Pharaoh's Oil - To evoke the power of empire and heritage of the gods.

Pharaoh's Dream - Prophetic dream concerning the welfare of the nation.

Pyramid Power - Mythical power generated at the center point of the pyramidal structure, said to preserve perishables indefinitely and grant great psychic and spiritual powers.

Ptah - God of Artisans, Artists, Designers, Builders and Metal Workers; Ancient creator of the Universe.

Qebusenuf - One of the four sons of Horus - Falcon headed God of the South - Canopic Guardian of the Intestines. Corresponding to the function of Assimilation and the element of fire.

Ra - Solar Deity, Ruler and Creator of the Gods.

Rait - Female counterpart of the god Ra.

Re - Variant of Ra.

Renemet - Goddess of Harvests and Suckling Babies who gave a baby its true name, personality and fate.

Renpet - Location of a shrine of Isis.

Sekhem - Variant name of Osiris.

Sefkhet-Seshat - Goddess of writing, letters, archives and surveyors; wife of Thoth; goddess of fate who measured the length of lives with palm branches.

Sekhmet - Lion headed goddess of war and healing; wife of Ptah; mistress of the demons of disease; avenging power of the sun.

Selket - Scorpion Goddess.

Seth - God of Chaos, Desert Storms, Barrenness, and Aridity, As Osiris and Horus personified the orderly civilization and life principle of the fertile regions of Egypt and of the Universe as a whole, Seth was their counterpart representing all the untamed forces that would overthrow that order.

Shai - God of Luck or Destiny.

Shait - Goddess of Destiny who traveled with the individual throughout life observing all the person's actions. When the soul was judged after death, it was Shait who gave the testimony.

Shetayet - Place of residence of an assessor called Basti.

Shezmu/Ashemu - The Great Power, God of Gods.

Shu - God of Air; first principle of the Life Force at the Creation of the Universe; Shu and his wife Tefnut were sometimes regarded as a pair of lions and also identified with the Akeru.

Sia - Counterpart of Hu, Companion of Ra, the personification of the knowledge and understanding of all things that made the Creation possible.

Sobek - Crocodile god of Fayum who was thought to have emerged from the Primordial Waters to lay the eggs of life on the shore.

Soped/Septu - War God "Smiter of the Asiatics".

Tait - One of the many names under which Hathor was worshipped.

Tauret/Ta-urt/Toueris - Ancient Hippopotamus goddess popularly worshipped along with Bes, protector of pregnant women and women in childbirth; one of the many animal forms of Mut the Great Mother.

Tchesert - Lake in the Land of the Blessed that cleansed away all dirt, sin, grief and pain.

Tefnut - Sometimes depicted as a lioness, Goddess of Atmospheric Moisture, i.e. rain dew, fog, principle of life potential at the Creation; along with her husband Shu identified as a lion and sometimes with the Akeru.

Thoth - God of Wisdom, Mathematics, Scribes, Magic, who gave writing to Humanity, overseer of the Moon because its cycles measured regular time, his animals were the ibis and the baboon.

Uajet - Sacred cobra goddess of Lower Egypt who along with Nekhbet the vulture goddess protected the Pharaoh.

Unnut - The Hare goddess, a protective goddess armed with knives.

Uraeus - Ancient form of the cobra goddess, protector of Lower Egyptian royalty, seen worn as the serpent band around the crown, also seen encircling the sun disk which crowns many solar associated deities as a manifestation of the solar eye, said to be the lightning striking power of the cobra which would strike down anyone who threatened or failed to tell the truth to the monarch.

Uto - Ancient snake goddess of Buto, connected with fertility and regeneration, later. Syncretized with Uajet, the protective cobra goddess of the monarchy.

Hindu Deities and Legendary Persons

Adibuddha - The concept of the Buddha that has existed from the beginning of time; the Buddha archetype.
Aditi - Infinity, The Great Goddess who rules the ordering of the world.
Adityas - The Eight Sons of Aditi, Celestial Deities, source of all heavenly gifts, regulator of all the forces of nature.
Agni - God of Fire and Lightning; mediator between gods and Humankind who carried the smoke of offerings and incense to the gods and departed souls to heaven.
Akupera - Goddess of Moonlight, daughter of Angiras, the spirit of fire as enlightenment.
Annapurna - Giver of Food and Plenty, One of the names of the Great Goddess.
Arjuna - Son of Indra, cousin of Krishna, warlike hero of the Mahabharata, favored by the gods with divine weapons.
Asuras, The - Demon enemies of the gods, who once lived in heaven and were expelled.
Asva - The horse that draws the Sun's Chariot.
Balarama - Ancient god of agriculture, older brother of Krishna.
Bhaga - God of fortune and prosperity, also god of marriage, one of the Aditayas.
Bhrigus, The - Shining ones; Aerial gods of lightning and storms who communicate between heaven and earth.
Brahma - Father of Gods and men, Creator of Heaven and Earth.
Brihaspati - Teacher of the gods, master of magic and created things who forwards the prayers of men to the ears of the gods, identified with the planet Jupiter.
Buddha - The Awakened One. The spirit of release from this Universe.
Buddha - Patron Spirit of the Planet Mercury.
Chandra - God of the Moon and source of fertility.
Dakini - Supernatural flying spirits in the Buddhist tradition who initiate Tantric apprentices in finding the hidden secrets.
Daksha - One of the Lords of Creation, father of Sati, Shiva's wife.
Dhanvantari - Physician of the gods and bearer of the gods' cup of the water of life.
Dharma - Duty, the means by which an individual accomplishes his or her Karma.
Dharme - God of the Path of Duty.
Diti - Goddess who grants wishes, daughter of Daksha.
Dyaus-Pitar - All father; sky god and father of the gods.

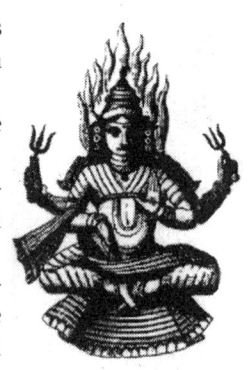

Gandharvas, The - Demigod spirits of nature and the atmosphere; Gods of the air, rain clouds and rain.
Ganesha - Elephant-headed son of Shiva and Parvati, Opener of Ways, Gods of Wisdom, Poetry, and all Worldly Prosperity.
Hanuman - Monkey god, patron of learning, renowned for his agility and speed.
Harihara - A composite twin deity, half-Shiva, half-Vishnu.
Himvat - God of the Himalayan Mountains, father of Parvati.
Indra - God of War, Lord of the Thunderbolt who brings rain.
Ishwara/Isvara - The universal concept of "God".
Jalandhara - A powerful demon who attempted to overthrow the gods and the divine order of creation; eventually Shiva conquered him with the aid of the goddesses.
Kali #1 - The Destroyer - Devouring goddess, fearful aspect of the Great Mother who frees her worshippers from all fears.
Kali #2 - The Creator - she devours all life at the end of their term to transform and transmute the life essence into new life; She who gives birth to the world from the death of the old.
Kalindi - Daughter of the Sun, one of Krishna's wives.
Kalki - Vishnu's tenth and last incarnation, he will appear at the end of the present age riding the horse, Kalki to destroy the world, preparing the way for a new Creation
Kamadeva - God of Love "Seed of Desire".
Kanya - The Virgin Aspect of the Great Mother.
Karttikeya - God of War.
Krishna - Heroic incarnation (8th) of Vishnu, god of erotic delight, skilled in warfare, prankster.
Kumari - Word meaning Princess.
Kundalini - The dormant energy coiled at the base of the spinal column that can be raised to focus great power for magic or other endeavors.
Kurma/Vishnu - Third avatar of Vishnu, the Turtle.
Lakshmi - Goddess of fortune and beauty - wife of Vishnu in all his avatars.
Lalita - Tantric goddess, symbol of universal cosmic energy and secret ruler of the world.
Lokapalas, The - Guardians of the compass points, Indra/East, Varuna/West, Yama/South, Kubera/North.
Lola - One of the names for the Goddess of Fortune meaning "the Fickle One".
Mahavira - Great teacher and founder of Jainism.
Manu - Creator of the human race.
Mari - Mother Goddess of the Dravidian peoples of southern India; goddess of rain; goddess of smallpox.
Maruts, The - Storm Spirits, the companions of Indra.
Matarisvan - Bringer of Fire to Mankind.

Maya - The female primeval principle by which the physical world was generated; the physical world; Goddess of Creativity.
Mayavati/Rati - "The Deceiver", Goddess of Passion, wife of Kama, God of Love
Mitra - God of Friendship and Contracts.
Naginis - Female serpent demons who sometimes look like nymphs, who sometimes haunt and terrorize rivers.
Narayana - The spirit of the first manifestation of Creation.
Parashurama - Sixth incarnation of Vishnu who broke the power of the warrior caste
Parjanya - Rain god, generator of vegetation.
Parvati - Wife of Shiva, Goddess of Marital Blessing, the image of the perfect wife and mother.
Prajapati - Creator who created himself out of the Primordial Waters.
Prajna - In Buddhism, the female principal; Intuition.
Radha - The cow-girl who was the beloved of Krishna.
Rama - Heroic seventh incarnation of Vishnu; he conquered the demon king of the Rakshas to rescue his wife Sita.
Ramachandra - Another name for Rama meaning "Rama of the Moon".
Rati - "The Deceiver", Goddess of Passion, wife of Kama, God of Love; Goddess of the passionate night, giver of rest, passion and regeneration.
Rukmini - Beautiful princess who became the first wife of Krishna.
Samadhya - Absolute focus and absorption in the object of that focus so that one is drawn out of the self and becomes the object.
Sambhuti - Fitness; one of the wives of the Seven Seers.
Saranyu - Goddess of Clouds.
Sarasvati - Wife of Brahma, Goddess of all Beauty and the Fine Arts.
Sarpis - Snake spirits; One of the race of semi-divinities called Maruts who are inhabitants of space that are worshipped to gain supernatural powers and for the fulfillment of ambitious projects.
Satarupa - Another name for Sarasvati, wife of Brahma.
Sati - The Good Wife; The focus name of many otherwise unnamed mother goddesses throughout India.
Shakti - Fulfillment; The female aspect of each god; Although the male aspects hold the power and potential of their attributes, it is only through their feminine counterparts that they are able to manifest them.
Shasti - Feline goddess who rides a lion; protector of childbirth and children.
Shitala - Goddess of smallpox; rides an ass, dressed in red, searching for victims.
Shiva - Great god of creation and generation who dances and with each step creates and destroys a Universe, weapon is a trident, wears the crescent moon on his forehead. Very ancient; worshipped by the Indus valley people before the coming of Vedic civilizations.

Shushumna - The forces that lead to suffering as the result of impure thoughts and ego directed impulses.

Sinvali - Giver of Fecundity, goddess of the first day of the new moon.

Sita - Wife of Rama who was abducted by the monkey king; After her rescue she walked through flames to prove her faithfulness and the flame did not burn her.

Soma - Moon god; Intoxicating drink that is the vital sap of all living creatures; The gods drink it from the moon bowl.

Sradda - Wife of the Manifestation of Fire (Angiras) whose name means Devotion.

Sri - One of the names of Lakshmi, Goddess of Fortune.

Sura - Goddess of Wine.

Surya - Sun god.

Tara - Her name means "She who delivers" and "Star"; supreme manifestation of the mother goddess; infinite of compassion and mercy; the name "Tara" is used as an epithet for most Hindu goddesses.

Trisald - Mother of Mahavira, dreamed prophetic dreams about her son's destiny.

Trita - One of the companions of the gods who consorts with the Gods of the atmosphere and with Agni prepares the Soma.

Urvasi - Beautiful nymph who so aroused Varuna and Surya that their "seed fell upon the ground"; This collected and gave birth to the great sage, Agastya.

Vishnu - Called "the Preserver" God who sustains the world, came into being in various forms called avatars nine times to save the world from chaos at the end of every great age, husband of Lakshmi.

Visvakarma - Brother of Indra, divine artisan, lord of smithcraft, lord of magic, maker of Indra's thunderbolts, archetype of the skilled craftsman.

Yama - God of the Dead; the first man to die.

Yami - The twin sister of Yama; together they were said to be the first man and woman.

Yatus - Magicians, sorcerers.

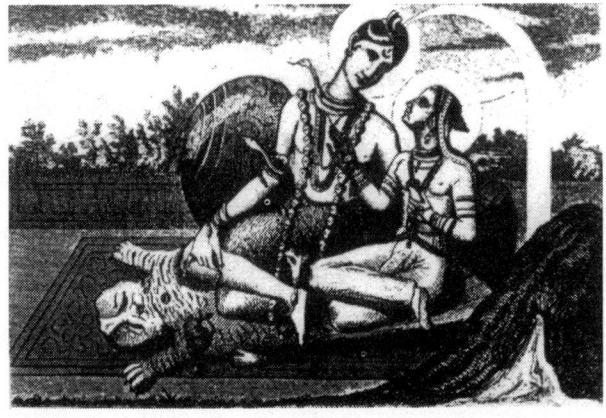

Mythical Creatures

Merman - Half man and half fish or dolphin, sometimes identified with the Selkie, one who is a man on land and turns into a seal in the ocean.

Mermaid - Half beautiful woman, half fish or dolphin, playful spirits of the waves and water, daughters of the King of the Sea.

Mermaid's Song - Unearthly, beautiful music that enchants sailors causing them to crash on the rocks and sink.

Nymph - A female wood spirit of great beauty and playfulness.

Phoenix - Magical fire bird who burst into flames that consumed it, then recreated itself and rose from its own ashes every thousand years.

Satyrs - Woodland spirit, half man, half-goat, spirits of the woodland wildness, known for their orgies and lechery.

Unicorn - Beautiful white creature with a single curling horn; sacred king incarnate in a horned horse that only a virgin can hold.

Mythical Places

Algiers - Exotic trade port of North Africa, city of mystery and intrigue.

Atlantis - Mythical island continent in the mid-Atlantic, seat of fabled wisdom and high technology that sank in a fiery volcanic explosion in three days time.

Babylon - Ancient city in the Tigris / Euphrates valley famous for its hanging gardens, exotic customs and wise men of learning.

Califa - Exotic power of an eastern queen.

Carmelite - Holy peace and sanctity of cloistered seclusion.

Mu - Island continent in the Pacific Ocean, predecessor of Atlantis, seat of ancient occult wisdom and fabled shape changing beast people.

Rainforest - Lush and beautiful tropical paradise, home of majestic trees, exquisite flora and magnificent animals.

Stonehenge - Astronomically oriented megalithic stone circle on the Salisbury Plain in England that is the focus of great power and energy.

Temple - Essence of a sacred sanctuary, consecrated and tuned to resonate to a high vibration. Enter its peace; partake of its energy.

Valhalla - Odin's hall where warriors slain in battle are brought by the Valkyries to feast, drink mead, party all night and fight to the death in battle all day.

Xanadu - "In Xanadu did Kublai Khan a stately pleasure dome decree" Create your private castle in the air.

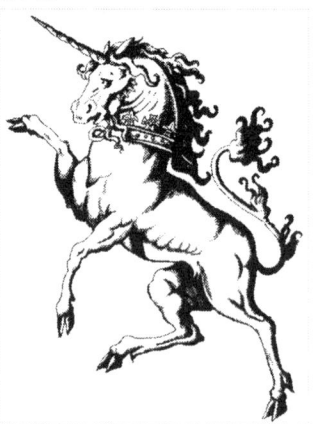

Norse Deities and Legendary Persons

Andavri - Dwarf who owned the treasure that Loki stole to pay the ransom for killing Otr.
Angurboda - "One who warns of danger", Giantess wife of Loki who gave birth to the Midgard Serpent, Fenris Wolf and the goddess Hel.
Audhumia - The divine cow who freed Bur, Odin's grandfather, from the Primordial Ice.
Baldur - Handsome and beloved son of Frigg and Odin who was killed by Loki's treachery.
Bragi - God of Poetry.
Brynhild - Shield maiden, female warrior who loved Sigurd (Sigfried).
Embla - First woman on Earth, fashioned by Odin from an Alder or Elm tree.
Erce - Slavic Earth mother honored every spring by pouring milk into the newly turned furrows.
Farbauti - "He who brings forth fire by striking", father of Loki.
Fjorgyn - Androgynous divinity who favors/gives life, a primordial deity of fecundity and fertility.
Frey - Son of Njord, the Sea God, whose name means "Lord" giver of sunshine and rain, peace, joy, fertility and relaxed happiness.
Freya - Goddess of Love, Beauty, Passion and War, Spirit of the Earth's fertility, rode a cat into battle.
Frigg - The heavenly matron, wife of Odin, goddess of all the wifely arts and virtues, dressed in hawk and falcon feathers.
Fulla - Abundance, fullness of the fruitful earth, handmaiden of Frigg.
Gerda - Goddess of light, beautiful giantess who lived in a house surrounded by fire and who shot flames from her hands, the most beautiful of creatures, wife of Frey.
Gerfjon - Virgin goddess, handmaiden of Frigg; patroness of virgins.
Heimdahl - Guardian of the rainbow bridge, Bifrost that led to Asgard, who will blow his horn to summon the gods to battle at the end of the world, Ragnarok.
Hela/Hel - Goddess who guarded the kingdom of the dead and determined where each soul would go, her hall was the abode of the souls who died of disease or illness.
Hlodyn/Jord - Daughter of night, Goddess of the primeval earth before mankind.
Hnossa - Goddess of Infatuation, Daughter of Freya, name means "Jewel".

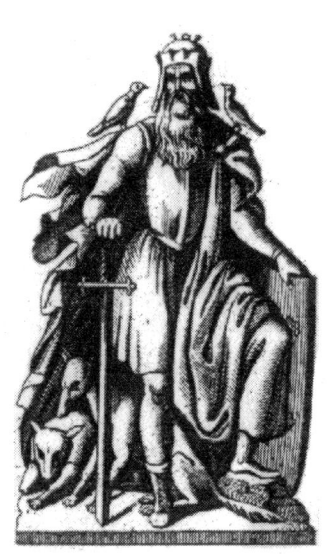

Hoenir/Heori - Giver of Humankind its sensibilities and senses; companion to Odin and Loki in their wanderings; renowned for his beauty, strength and boldness.

Hoder - Blind god tricked by Loki into killing Baldur by throwing a sprig of mistletoe at him.

Holda/Hulda - Ancient Mother Goddess personified as a stone with a natural hole in it. This was said to be the gateway between the worlds through which she would whisper her secrets to her initiates.

Iduna - Goddess of Youth and Strength, keeper of the magic apples that were the only food of the gods without which they would weaken, starve and die.

Jorth - Another name for Hlodwyn - Goddess of the Primeval Earth.

Lodehur - Giver of Humankind its Life force and fresh color.

Loki - God of Mischief, Magician, Shape-shifter, Trickster par excellence.

Mimir - God of Wisdom; the waters from his spring water the world tree and were said to give the drinker all knowledge.

Nanna - Quiet and beautiful wife of Baldur, who shared his funeral pyre out of grief for him.

Nixes - Prophetic spirits of the waters, river mermaids.

Njord - God of the Sea and Ships.

Norns, The - Nurturers of the world tree, goddesses of each person's fate/destiny who taught the individual life's rules. The individual's luck depended on the skill of his Norn. Later identified with the Three Great Norns who, like the Greek Fates, ruled the Past, Present and Future.

Odin - All-Father; One-eyed god of battle, death and inspiration, God of wisdom who hung nine days on the world tree to gain the knowledge of the runes, creator of humankind.

Ran - Great Sea Goddess, Queen of the drowned, sailors carried gold on their person to bribe their way into her hall, great mermaid, lover of gold.

Saga - All knowing goddess, second only to Frigg, name means "Omniscience".

Sif - Grain goddess whose golden hair was the autumn grass, lived with Thor.

Sin - Fairy woman who turned water into wine and leaves into pigs to feed to her magical host of warriors.

Sjofna - Handmaiden of Frigg who stirred infatuation in human hearts.

Skadi - Mountain goddess who married the sea god, Njord, but was unhappy with him. She later left him to return to her mountain home and married Uller, god of skiing and archery.

Thor - God of Thunderstorms and fertility, Giver of marital happiness, protector of herds and crops, His weapon was the great thunder hammer, Mjolnir.

Ullur - Administer of Justice, God of Archery, Snow shoes and Skiing.

Vainamoinen - legendary Finnish hero, bard and shaman.

Vali - Son of Odin and Rind who avenged the death of Baldur by slaying Hoder.

Ve - Brother of Villi and Odin, together they slew the giant Ymir and made the earth from his bones and the sea from his blood.

Vidar - Son of Odin "the Silent One" he hardly ever spoke but when he stamped his foot, all the world would listen, slayer of Fenris Wolf at Ragnarok; survivor of the last battle who would live to regenerate the world.

Woden - Germanic version of Odin.

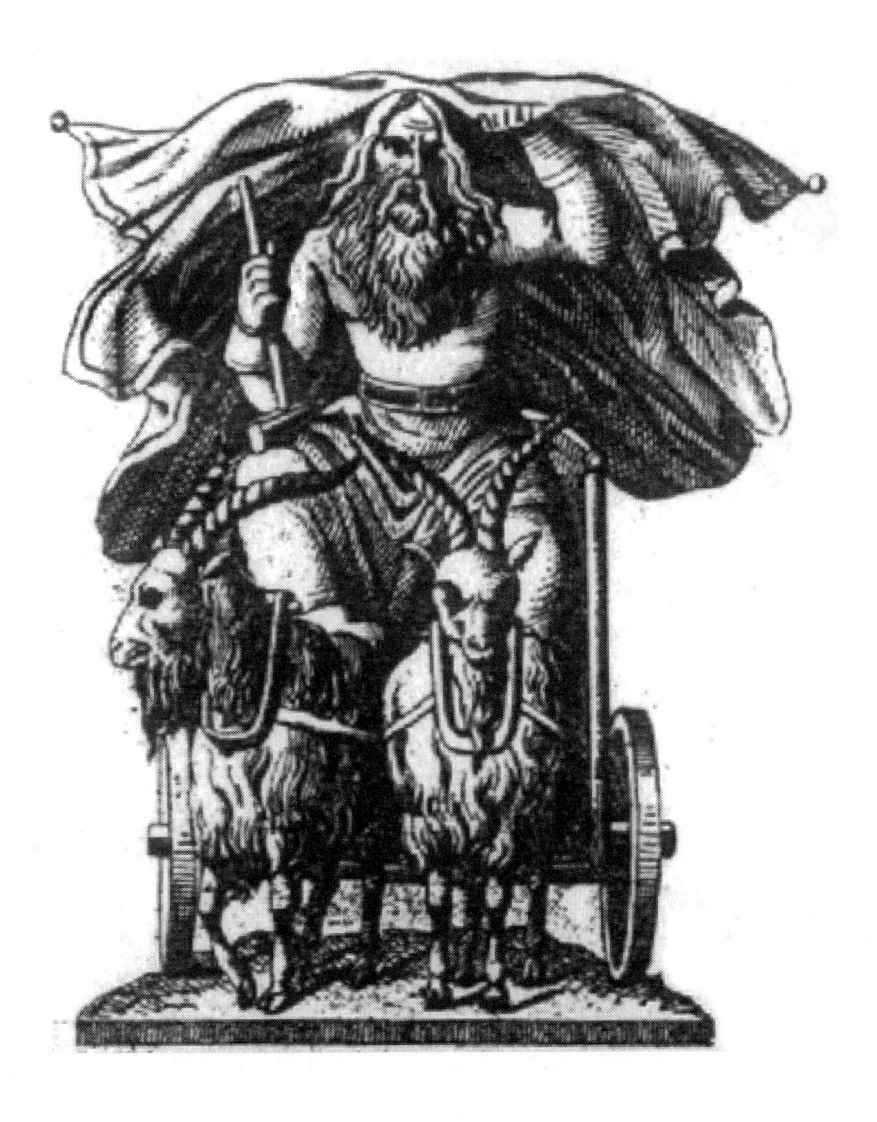

Greco-Roman Deities and Legendary Persons

Achelous - River god; oldest son of Tethys and Oceanus; father of the Sirens.
Adonis - Beautiful youth loved by Aphrodite, killed by a wild boar and from his blood sprang the anemone. See also Tammuz, Damuzi.
Adraste - Goddess of Destiny, of the Inevitable, Nemesis.
Andromeda - Princess of Joppa chained to a rock to appease Poseidon; rescued by Perseus; turned into a constellation by Athena.
Aphrodite - Goddess of Love, Beauty and Pleasure.
Apollo - Sun God, also god of Fine Arts, Music, Poetry, Healing and Prophecy.
Ares - God of War.
Artemis - Moon goddess, Virgin huntress goddess, protector of unmarried women, virgin girls, the young of all animals.
Astraea - Roman goddess of Justice; became the constellation Virgo.
Athena - Daughter of Zeus; goddess of wisdom and warfare.
Atlanta - Heroine of the Caledonian boar hunt; ran a foot race against all her suitors, the one who won to marry her, but Hippomenes won her by throwing Aphrodite's golden apple at her feet so that he won the race when she stopped to pick it up.
Atlas - One of the Titans who carried the earth and all the heavens on his shoulders.
Cadmos - Hero; Builder of the city of Thebes, brought the use of letters to Greece.
Callisto - Mistress of Zeus who was changed into the constellation, The Great Bear, (the Big Dipper) Their son Arcos was changed into the Small Bear (the Little Dipper).
Cassiopeia - Mother of Andromeda who angered Poseidon by bragging that she was more beautiful than his daughter. Became a constellation.
Castor - (and his twin brother Pollux) Sons of Zeus and Leda; heroes who became the constellation Gemini; Castor became a famous horseman.
Charon - Boatman who ferried the souls of the dead across the River Styx to Hades.
Circe - Daughter of Apollo and Perseis, Enchantress, mistress of magic & herbs, lover of Odysseus, turned his men into swine.
Cronus - Titan synonymous with Roman Saturn, God of Time.
Cybele/Rhea - The Titan Earth Goddess, daughter of Gaia, wife of Chronus.
Cyclopes - Three one eyed giant monsters; sons of the Titans.

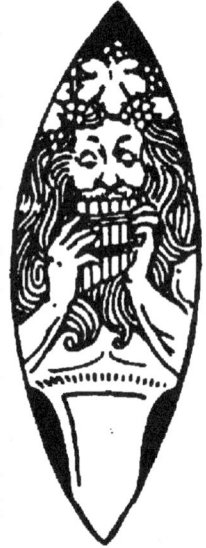

Delphi Oracle - Sanctuary of Apollo where the priestess gave prophesy.
Demeter - Goddess of Agriculture, Fertility, Guardian of Marriage; Mother of Plutus, god of wealth.
Diana - Another name for the Moon Goddess, Artemis.
Dionysus - God of Wine, Revelry and Ecstasy.
Electra - She and her brother, Orestes, killed their mother Clytemnestra, to avenge their father, Agamemnon's death and were hounded to death by the Harpies.
Erebus - Son of Darkness and Chaos, one of the guardians of the Underworld the dead must pass on their way to judgment.
Eros - God of passionate love.
Europa - Mistress of Zeus, mother of Minos, King of Crete, by Zeus.
Evenor - Grandmother of the five successive pairs of twins who ruled Atlantis.
Hades - King of the Underworld.
Harmonia - Wife of Cadmos, daughter of Ares and Aphrodite, some say mother of the Amazons.
Helios - Another name for Apollo in his role as the sun god.
Hephaestos - God of Fire and Smithcraft.
Hera - Wife of Zeus, Patroness of Women and childbirth, Mistress of Gods and Heaven.
Hercules - Legendary hero of enormous strength.
Hermes - Roman Mercury, messenger of the gods, god of trade and travelers, god of wealth and increase in the animal world, trickster, thief.
Hestia - Virgin Goddess of the Hearth and symbol of the home.
Hyperion - Another name for Apollo Helios.
Hypnos - God of Sleep, father of Morpheus, god of dreams.
Iris - Goddess of the rainbow, messenger of the gods.
Ladon - The dragon that guarded the apples of the Hesperides, the garden owned by Atlas.
Medea - Powerful enchantress, wife of Jason who helped him win the Golden fleece by killing her brother.
Medusa - One of the three gorgons who had the power to turn to stone anyone who looked on their faces.
Minos - King of Crete, son of Zeus and Europa who had the inventor Daedalus build the Labyrinth to house the Minotaur.
Morpheus - God of dreams.
Nemesis - Goddess of Vengeance.
Nymph - A female wood spirit of great beauty, often wives and mistress of the greater gods.
Orion - Legendary hero and hunter whom Artemis placed in the heavens as a constellation.
Pan - Part man, part goat, lascivious and lecherous, playful; god of flocks and herds, forests and wild life, patron of shepherds and hunters.
Pandora - Curious mortal who was given a sealed box to keep, her curi-

osity overcame her and when she opened the box, all the troubles of the world flew out of it, leaving only hope.

Pegasus - Magical winged horse; symbol of poetic inspiration.

Persephone - Daughter of Demeter, Queen of the Underworld, wife of Hades who causes winter by living in the underworld half the year.

Perseus - Hero, rescuer and husband of Andromeda, slayer of Medusa, founder of Mycenae and Tiryns.

Phoebe - Titan; first moon goddess before Artemis.

Poseidon - Great god of the sea, brother of Zeus.

Prometheus - Defied the gods to give fire to mankind.

Psyche - Name means "soul", married Eros, god of Love.

Rhea - Titan earth goddess, wife of Chronos, Great mother goddess, mother of many of the Olympians.

Sappho - Lyric poetess born on the Island of Lesbos, credited with lesbian love poems

Satyrs - Sylvan deities, half man, half-goat, attendants of Dionysus (some say of Pan), spirits of the woodland wildness, known for their orgies and lechery.

Selene - Another name for the Moon goddess, Artemis.

Triton - Son of Poseidon, half fish or dolphin, powerful sea deity; later a name for any merman.

Ulysses (Roman form of Odysseus) - Hero designer of the Trojan horse; famous for his caution, intelligence, and quick wit having offended the gods at the fall of Troy, he wandered for twelve years before being allowed to return home.

Zeus - Ruler of Heaven and Earth of all the Gods and all Humankind.

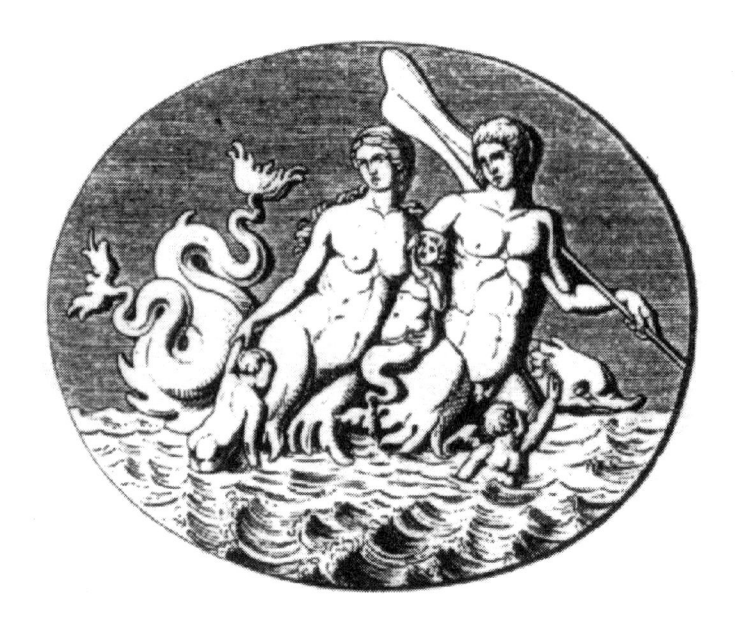

Oriental Wisdom

Buddha - The Awakened One, The spirit of release from this Universe.

I Ching - A Chinese method of divination by the drawing of yarrow sticks or tossing of coins. The combination of coin faces describing a combination of 6 broken or solid lines whose pattern indicates which of 64 passages in the I Ching or Book of Changes is applicable to the question at hand.

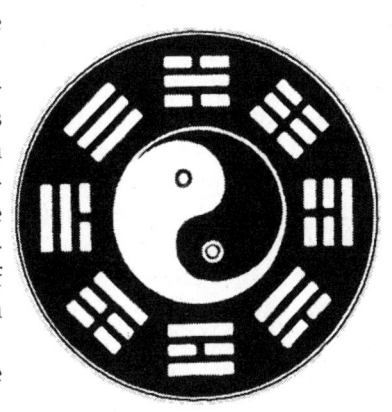

Kwan-Yuen - Goddess of Infinite Mercy & Compassion.

Lingam - Male genitalia as a symbol of the absolute male active generative principle.

Nirvana - Buddhist state of non-being; the state at which no Karmic interactives are in motion. Freedom from the wheel of Karma and from the bonds of the physical universe.

Samurai - One who follows the Path of Bushido, the path of obedience and discipline of a warrior.

Tibetan Meditation - The sound of ringing prayer bowls carry the spirit outward; union with the source of all things.

Tibetan Prayer - Resonance of ancient invocations drawing ages old earth and sky forces through elegant Buddhist liturgy.

Yang - One of the opposite poles of existence in the Universe representing active, aggressive, male, light, heat elements.

Yin - One of the opposite poles of existence in the Universe representing, passive, receptive, female, dark, cool elements.

Yin & Yang - The union and balance of the two opposing states in the duality of the universe each containing a part of the other, sometimes represented as the balance and harmony of male and female together.

Yoni - Female genitalia as a symbol of the absolute feminine creative life force.

Zen - Tranquil path of peace and simplicity.

Shamanic

Allies - Draw & awaken to your animal spirit guides and helpers.
Bear Spirit - Strength through spiritual Attunement, mother strength of the tribe.
Buffalo Dancer - Move to the rhythm of the earth and the flow of the Universe, learn to draw abundance of life and heart.
Buffalo Spirit - Prayer and abundance come as a result of oneness with the earth and the flow of life.
Cougar Spirit - Visionary leadership of the spiritual, mystical cat, march to the beat of your own drummer.
Coyote Spirit - The trickster, learning to laugh at ourselves, coyote plays tricks that teach us about our most basic shortcomings.
Crow Spirit - Keeper of the sacred law, shape-changer; knower of the ancient wisdom, omen of change.
Dolphin Spirit - Joyful ocean spirit of love, peace and play, at one with the sun and waves.
Dream Catcher - Catches dreams as they come from the spirit world, traps the bad ones only letting through the happy ones or ones you need for information.
Eagle Spirit - Spirit messenger from Great Spirit, power to rise above yourself to do great things, magnificent cloud rider.
Eagle Woman - The words of spirits speak through her - her heart opens and spirit flows through her giving her visions to bring to her people and strength to do great things.
Eagle's Flight - Brings the wisdom of the Great Spirit to the people, takes the prayers of the people to the heavens.
Elk Spirit - Endurance, strength of heart, to outlast the pursuer.
Fire Dance - Dance of passion and power, give yourself over to the magnetic and empowering spirit of the flames, they dance through your soul bringing joy and release.
Fox Spirit - Invisibility, adaptability, learn from all you see, be wily, aware, to take care of your own.
Hawk Spirit - Messenger from the spirit world, time to pay attention.
Father Sky - He who shelters and protects his children, gives us sun and rain in season and time.
Great Spirit - Flowing consciousness that moves throughout all creation and all time.
Lynx Spirit - Knower of secrets, teaches the inner knowledge of the heart and self.

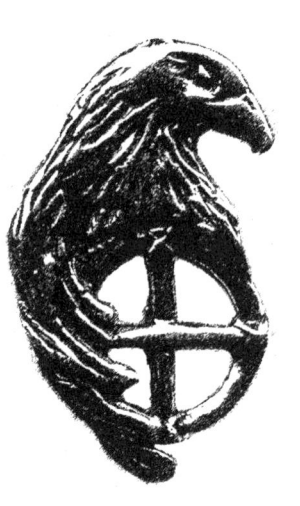

Medicine Man - Knower of animals and herbs. Helps the people be whole in body and spirit.

Moon Dancer - Move with the flow of natural changes - feel the silvery light and the rhythms of the night.

Mother Earth - Gave birth to all Creation, who loves and nurtures her children.

Northwind - Cooling wind of wisdom, road of the ancestors.

Owl Spirit - Spirit that finds truth seeing what others cannot see; silent hunter of the twilight, the time between times, neither day nor night; the place between the worlds.

Raven Spirit - Spirit of the battle field who flies between the worlds of the living and the world of the spirits; bird of secrets and purpose.

Prairie Song - Feel the freedom and spiritual expansion of the wind as it blows through the sun warmed tall grasses - song of life and plenty.

Shaman - Walks between the many worlds to learn and bring back magic and wisdom.

Shaman's Dream - The message comes in the night, cryptic message to bring growth and illumination.

Shaman's Journey - The seeking spirit travels into the underworld to bring back the knowledge of power and healing.

Shaman's Vision - The spirit opens to receive a message from spirit guides and totem helpers in answer to the Shaman's quest.

Shape-Shifter - Magically adaptable at will; take the essence of your totem inside you, let it come through you to reveal your inner nature.

Smudge - Cleansing and purifying; the sacred herbs cleanse the heart and spirit preparing the space for meditation, worship or living.

Snake Spirit - Spirit of regeneration and rebirth, spirit of flow moving over and around obstacles.

Spider Spirit - Weaver of dreams, weavers of worlds, weaver of fate on the wheel of life.

Spirit Dancer - Power and passion fill the heart with the rhythm of the flow of the universe, feel it move you and move through you.

Sundance - Opening the self to spirit, through trial and triumph the Seeker is cleansed and filled with the light of spirit.

Tirawa - Pawnee - The power that has ordered all things and gives all creatures everything they need.

Turtle Spirit - Grounded and sturdy foundation, shield and protection, firm stance of strength.

Wolf Spirit - Clan medicine, pack brotherhood, explorer, leader into the unknown.

Shamanic Essential Fragrances

Cedar - Calming and comforting scent with strength to purify and protect.
Juniper - Cleansing and centering, brings clarity and focus.
Lemongrass - Tonic and refreshing, stimulates the inner connection with spirit opening the channel to inner voices and higher wisdom.
Pine - Strengthening and cleansing, opens the way for regeneration and expansion.
Sage - Balancing and strengthening, cleanses the spirit so that peace and wisdom may enter, banishes negativity.
Sweetgrass - "Indian Incense" calls and opens the way for spirit helpers and higher wisdom.

Choose the combination that best suits your magical and spiritual purpose:

Cedar & Sage	Lemongrass & Pine	Sage & Lemongrass
Cedar & Sweetgrass	Sage & Sweetgrass	Juniper & Cedar
Pine & Sage	Sweetgrass & Juniper	Juniper & Pine
Sage & Juniper	Wildflowers	

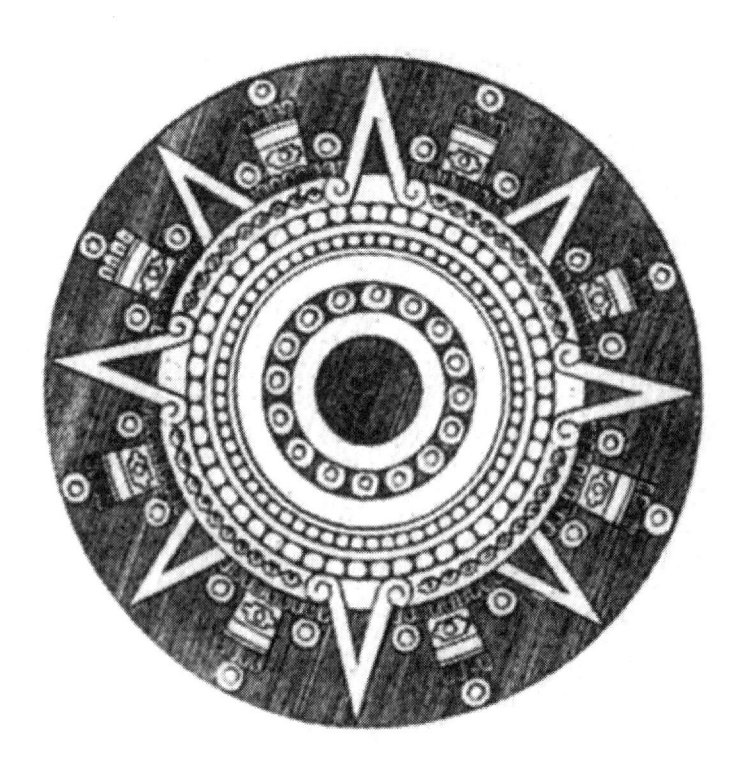

Welsh Deities and Legendary Persons

Amaethon - One of the sons of Don, God of Agriculture

Arawma - King in the Underworld who appealed to Pwyll for help

Arianrhod - Wildflowers Moon goddess whose name means "Silver Wheel" or "High Fruitful Mother", daughter of Don, mother of Llew Llaw Gyffes and Dylan

Avagduv - Ugliest man in the world, son of Ceridwen, for who the gift of supernatural insight was intended, that was taken by accident, instead by Gwion.

Beli/Belenus - Solar & Fire god brought life fire to all creatures

Blodeuwedd - Wife of Llew Llaw Gyffes made from flowers by his uncle Gwydion

Bran - One of the ancient Guardians of Britain, Son of Llyr

Branwen - Sister of Bran the Blessed, one of the three matriarchs of Britain

Caradawg - Son of Bran who ruled the British Isles in his father's absence

Caswallawn - Son of Beli, usurped the Isle of Britain and drove out the sons of Llyr

Ceridwen - Keeper of the Cauldron of Knowledge, Inspiration and Rebirth

Creiddylad/Cordelia - Sea Queen - Daughter of Llyr whose suitors, Gwythyr and Greidawl must fight each other every May Day until Doomsday

Culhwch - Mortal husband of Olwen, the Sun Goddess

Don/Danu - Mother of the Great Gods of the Tuatha da Dannan

Dwyvan - God of love, the "Welsh Cupid", son of the Dagda, brother of Brigit

Dylan - "Son of the Wave", a sea god, son of Arianrhod

Goleuddydd - Wife of Killyd, mother of the hero Kilhwch

Govannon - God of Smithcraft & Brewing, son of Don

Gronw Pebr - Lover of Bloddeuwed who conspired with her to kill her husband, Llew Llaw Gyffes

Gwion - Servant of Ceridwen who drank three drops from her cauldron of All Knowledge. In anger she devoured him but later gave birth to him as Taliesin the great bard

Gwydion - Magician, bard, god of civilization, brother of Arianrhod

Gwyn - Son of Nuada, Warder of Hades

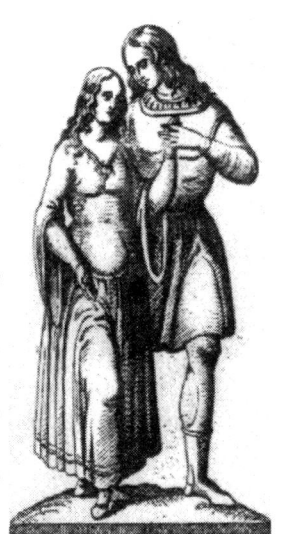

Hu-Gadarm - (Hu the Mighty) - Welsh hero who brought knowledge of

the plow and the skill of using song as an aid to memory

Idrasa - Giant said to be able to foretell the future by the stars; whoever spends a night on his mountain will be either inspired or mad by morning

Iseult - Wife of King Marc of Cornwall who abandoned him for her lover Tristan

Llew Llaw Gyffes - Son of Arianrhod, god of brightness and the sun's shining face, "Sure Hand" of the true aim, murdered by his wife & her lover, brought back by his uncle

Llyr - Sea god, son of Don

Mabon - Son of Modron, huntsman who must aid Kilwch in hunting the great boar Twrch Trwyth, one of the tasks to winning the hand of Olwen

Manawyddan - God of the Ocean Depths, holder of fantastic treasure, son of Don

Math ap Mathonwy - God of Sorcery, son of Don

Myrddin - Chieftain god of the Underworld

Modron - Mother of Mabon the Huntsman

Olwyn - Welsh Sun Goddess "Golden Wheel", "White Lady of the Day"; daughter of Ysbadden who was sought by the hero Kilhwch

Pryderi - Son of Pwyll who succeeded to the Kingship of the Underworld on his father's passing

Pwyll - Prince of Annwn, the Welsh Underworld, married Rhiannon

Rhiannon - Goddess of Birds, Underworld Goddess - also Rigantona "Great Queen"

Taliesin - Legendary Welsh bard and mage, son of Ceridwen

Tristan - Hero of courtly love tradition, wizard, poet, dragon slayer, lover of Queen Iseult

Ysbadaddenv - Father of Olwen who set Kilhwch many supernatural tasks to win the hand of his daughter

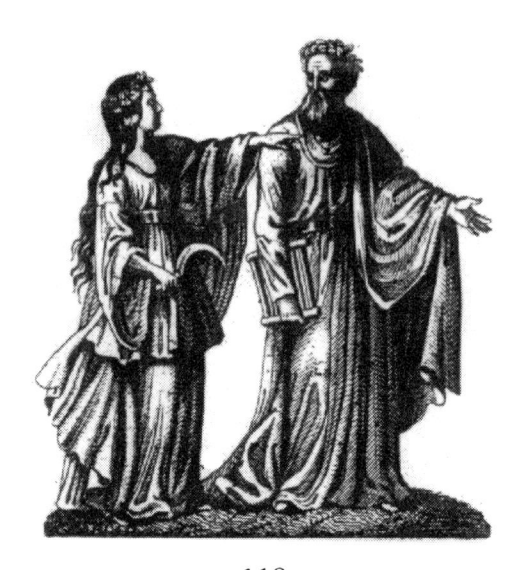

Wiccan Archetypes

Air Child - One who is gifted with the blessings of quick speech, light laughter, communication, agility - a sylph like, fairy like person.

Baphomet - Bisexual idol or talking head worshipped by the Templars as a source of wisdom.

Earth Child - One who is gifted with the blessings of solidity, abundance, practicality, and endurance - a maker of things - a gnome-like person.

Enchanter - Male who weaves a magical spell on another person.

Enchantress - Female who weaves a magical spell on another person.

Father Sky - The father principle, he who shelters and protects his children, who gives us sun and rain in season and time.

Fire Child - One who is gifted with the blessings of passion, joy, action, energy - a salamander -like person.

God - The archetypal male deity principle of the universe who has all names and no name.

Goddess - The archetypal female deity principle of the universe who has all names and no name.

Green Man - The personification of wild life and spring, the spirit of vigorous earth life wild consciousness in all things.

Hecate - Queen of Night, the Dark Moon Goddess, crone aspect worshipped at the crossroads, Greek name for the threefold goddess trinity ruler of heaven, earth and the underworld; Queen of the Ghost World hence, Queen of Witches.

Holly King - The winter god/king - the ever living immortal spirit of vegetation and life who stands green and unfaded even in the midst of winter symbolizing life that exists undiminished even after seeming death.

Horned God - The hunter, the god of nature, the son/lover of Mother Earth; impregnator and fertilizer of Mother Earth; lord of the dance to the rhythms of life, death and rebirth.

Lady of the Night - Lady of Dreams and Secrets, of lovers' meetings.

Lady of the Woods - Lady of Vegetation of the Wild Places, animal mother, tree spirit.

Lord - The male deity principle as manifested on this plane in this world - Creator, father, hunter, warrior, lover, brother, child.

Magus - One wisdom and highly learned in the arts of magic.

Moon Goddess - The goddess in her aspects as symbolized by the phases of the Moon - the goddess as the Maiden symbolized by the waxing moon, Mother symbolized by the full moon, and the Crone symbolized by the waning moon.

Mother Earth - The Earth Goddess, Bona Dea, She who gave birth to all Creation and who loves and nurtures her children.

Oak King - The summer god/king - The symbol of summer vegetation and abundance that yearly dies to be reborn the following year.

Old Man of the Woods - The Wild Man - the spirit of the wild animal nature in resident in all living creatures, spirit of the woodland wilds, spirit of fertility, fecundity and abandon in the manner of Pan and the Satyrs.

Pagani - The Italian word for rural country people who kept the old ways and religion alive through the centuries and from which the word pagan derives.

Queen of the Stars - Aspect of the Goddess picture with her body as the Milky Way.

Sorcerer - Male who works magic to achieve an end and control the physical world.

Sorceress - Female who works magic to achieve an end and control the physical world.

Sun God - The god as seen in the solar aspect, sky father, the light bringer.

Three Ladies - The Triple goddess the goddess as seen in her three aspects as the Maiden, the Mother, and the Crone.

Water Child - One who is gifted with the blessings of intuition, dreams, fluidity, grace, coolness, a mermaid or undine-like person.

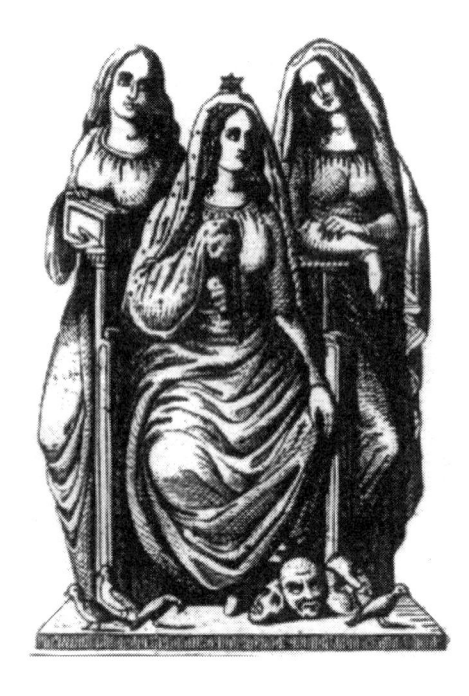

Bibliography

Ardinger, Barbara, A Woman's Book of Rituals and Celebrations, New World Library, San Raphael, CA : 1992

Barber, Richard, A Companion to World Mythology, Delacorte Press, New York: 1979

Beyerl, Paul, The Master Book of Herbalism, Phoenix Publishing, Custer, WA: 1984

Bonefoy, Yves, comp. Mythologies, 2 volumes, trans. Wendy Doniger, University of Chicago Press, Chicago: 1991.

Book of Saints, compiled by the Benedictine Monks of St. Augustine's Abbey, Ramsgate (6th Edition) Morehouse Publishing, Wilton, CT: 1989

Budge, E. A. Wallis, Gods of the Egyptians, Vols. 1 & 2, Dover Publications, New York: 1969

Carlyon, Richard, A Guide to the Gods, Quill, New York: 1982

Case, Paul Foster, The Tarot, a Key to the Wisdom of the Ages, Builders of the Adytum, Los Angeles: 1990

Culpeper, Nicholas, Culpeper's Complete Herbal, W. Foulsham & Co, Ltd, New York: 1971

Cunningham, Scott, Cunningham's Encyclopedia of Magickal Oils, Llewellyn Publications, St. Paul, MN: 1992

Danielou, Paul, The Gods of India, Inner Traditions International, New York: 1985

Davidson, Gustav, A Dictionary of Angels, The Free Press, New York: 1967

Farrar, Janet & Stewart, The Witches' God, Phoenix Publishing, Custer, WA: 1989

Fischer-Rizzi, Susanne, Complete Aromatherapy Handbook: Essential Oils for Radiant Health, Sterling Publishing Co., New York: 1990

Fitch, Ed., Magical Rites from the Crystal Well, Lewellyn Publications, St. Paul, MN: 1984

Goodrich, Norma Lorre, The Ancient Myths, Mentor Books, New York: 1960

_____, Medieval Myths, Mentor Books, New York: 1961

George, Llewellyn, A to Z Horoscope Maker and Delineator, Llewellyn Publications, St. Paul, MN:1975

_____, Improved Perpetual Planetary Hour Book, Llewellyn Publications, St. Paul, MN: 1975

Greer, Mary Katherine, The Essence of Magic, Newcastle Publishing, North Hollywood, CA: 1993

Grimal, Pierre., Ed, The Larousse World Mythology. Hamlyn Publishing Group Ltd. London:1989

Gundarsson, Kveldulf, Teutonic Religion, Folk Beliefs and Practices of the Northern Tradition, Llewellyn Publications, St. Paul, MN: 1993

Hamilton, Edith, Mythology, Mentor Books, New York: 1962

Huson, Paul, Mastering Herbalism, Stein and Day, New York: 1974
Hutton, Ronald, Pagan Religions of the British Isles, Blackwell Publishers, Oxford: 1992
Ions, Veronica, Indian Mythology, Paul Hamlyn Ltd., London: 1967
Lacey, Norris J., Ed., The New Arthurian Encyclodepia, Garland Publishing Co., New York: 1991
Lurker, Manfried, Dictionary of Gods & Goddesses, Devils & Demons, Routeledge and Kegan Paul, London and New York: 1987
MacCullough, Canon John Arnoti, Editor, The Mythology of All Races in Thirteen Volumes, Cooper Square Publishers, Inc., New York: 1964
Monaghan, Patricia. The Book of Goddesses and Heroines, Elsevier-Dutton Publishing Co., New York: 1981
Omarr, Sidney, My World of Astrology, Wilshire Book Company, No. Hollywood, CA: 1970
Rolleston, T. W., Myths & Legends of the Celtic Race, Schoken Books, New York: 1986
Rose, Jeanne, The Aromatherapy Book, North Atlantic Books, Berkeley, CA: 1992
Sams, Jamie and David Carson, Medicine Cards, Bear & Company Publishing, Santa FE, NM: 1988
Schumacher, Stephan and Gert Woerner, Editors., The Encyclopedia of Eastern Philosophy and Religion, Shambala, Boston: 1989.
Sun Bear and Wabun, The Medicine Wheel, Earth Astrology, Prentice Hall Inc., Englewood. NJ: 1980
Vinci, Leo, Incense, Its Ritual Significance, Use and Preparation, Samuel Weiser, New York: 1980
Waite, Arthur Edward, The Pictorial Key to the Tarot, Harper & Row, San Francisco, CA: 1971
Williamson, John, The Oak King, the Holly King and the Unicorn. Harper and Row, New York: 1986
Zimmerman, J. E. Dictionary of Classical Mythology, Bantam Books, New York: 1966

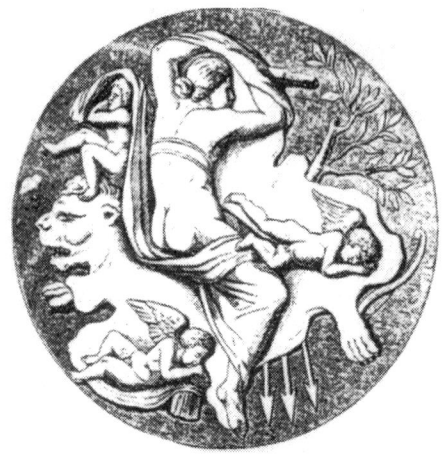

About the Author

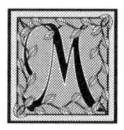

Maya Heath was born in Denton, Texas, on March 24, 1948. She studied theology, theater, literature, and linguistics at the University of Houston graduating in 1971. Her lifelong passion for art and ancient history has gone hand-in-hand with her deep and abiding interest in metaphysics and higher consciousness studies. She has appeared on television and radio and has lectured and taught on metaphysics, energy and crystal work, self-hypnosis and magic. She is the author of The Egyptian Oracle and the forthcoming Energies. If you or your organization would like information personal appearances, lectures, and workshops your correspondence may be addressed to:

Maya Heath
P.O. Box 12212
Parkville, MO 64152-0212

or via Electronic mail:
dragonscal@aol.com

The author welcomes your questions and comments on this work and will make every attempt to answer correspondence that she receives. However, due to her schedule and the volume of correspondence this may not always be possible, but, she thanks you for your time and interest.

About the Cover Artist

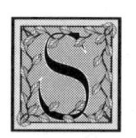

Steve Goins is an artist of exceptional versatility and vision. He allows information to create images without interjection of ego, which can be seen in the pictures, jewelry, eggs, spheres and drums he uses as a vehicle of transportation for the images translated. Steve can be contacted at :Thought Transition, 2704 NW 26th Street, OKC, OK 73107 (405) 946-8205

About Ceridwen's

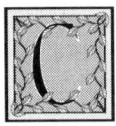

Ceridwen's Magical & New Age Supplies began in Los Angeles in 1985 as the ripening fruit of Sharon Helton's lifetime association with the world of spirits. Since early childhood, Sharon has been in contact with many spirits who played important roles in the shaping of her life. As a young adult, Sharon traveled from Australia to England to study in the Spiritualist Church and learn more about her native gift. A short time after moving to the USA, she began using her insight and talents to help others understand and deal with their lives. When people started asking for charms to help them achieve desired changes, Sharon began mixing "Herbal Helpers". Many of her spirit friends gifted her with recipes for oils and incenses feeling they would benefit people everywhere. Zeus in particular charged her with making "Oils for Mankind". Sharon dedicated her budding business to Ceridwen, mate of the Celtic god Cernunnos, who together stir the cauldron of rebirth. With the blessings of Ceridwen, and her own lifelong desire to help people, Sharon built the business into an international supplier of herbs, incenses, fragrant oils and other products, one of the largest in the country.

In 1993, Sharon sold Ceridwen's, with all her original recipes, to Bob Isaac, owner of Merlin's Books and Gifts in Independence, Missouri, who continues the tradition of excellence and dedication to helping others with which this company was created and nurtured.

Ceridwen's Magickal & New Age Supplies

630 S. Huttig
Independence, MO 64053
USA (816) 461-7773
Monday thru Saturday 10 am to 7 pm CST

The oils, incense, and bath crystals you have seen described here are all available from Ceridwen's Magical & New Age Supplies based in Independence Missouri since 1993.

Ceridwen's is one of the largest occult, spiritual and New Age suppliers in the country. We're large enough to serve you promptly and efficiently, with the finest quality products and personal service. All the oils and incense in this book are original recipes whose properties have been tested over the years by Ceridwen's customers.

We carry a full line of magickal and metaphysical supplies and will be happy to send a mail order catalogue upon request People report many positive results that they associate with the use of Ceridwen's products. All our products are sold as curios only. We make no claims nor guarantee of supernatural or magickal qualities for any item. Names and alleged powers are drawn from books, folklore and various occult and historical sources.

Copyright Notice

All recipes and formula names appearing in this work are the property of Ceridwen's Magical, Metaphysical & New Age Supplies and may not be copied or used in any way, except by express written permission. Ceridwen's Handbook of Incense Oils and Candles © 1996 Robert B. Isaac. All parts reserved, no part of this publication may be reproduced by any means or in any way whatsoever without written permission from the publisher, except for brief quotations embodied in literary articles or reviews. Some Interior Illustrations Copyright 1996 Wade Berlin, Portions Copyright 1996 Ancient Pathways Corp., used with Permission.